John H. Thompson

The diseases and injuries of the conjunctiva

Especially the so-called granulated lids

John H. Thompson

The diseases and injuries of the conjunctiva
Especially the so-called granulated lids

ISBN/EAN: 9783742805638

Manufactured in Europe, USA, Canada, Australia, Japa

Cover: Foto ©Lupo / pixelio.de

Manufactured and distributed by brebook publishing software
(www.brebook.com)

John H. Thompson

The diseases and injuries of the conjunctiva

THE
Diseases and Injuries
OF THE
Conjunctiva,

Especially the
So-Called Granulated Lids.

BY

JOHN H. THOMPSON, M.D.
Professor of Ophthalmology and Otology, Kansas City Medical
College, Kansas City, Mo.

———————

FIRST EDITION,
(With Illustrations.)

———————

KANSAS CITY, MO.
HUDSON-KIMBERLY PUBLISHING CO.
1014-1016 WYANDOTTE STREET.
1897.

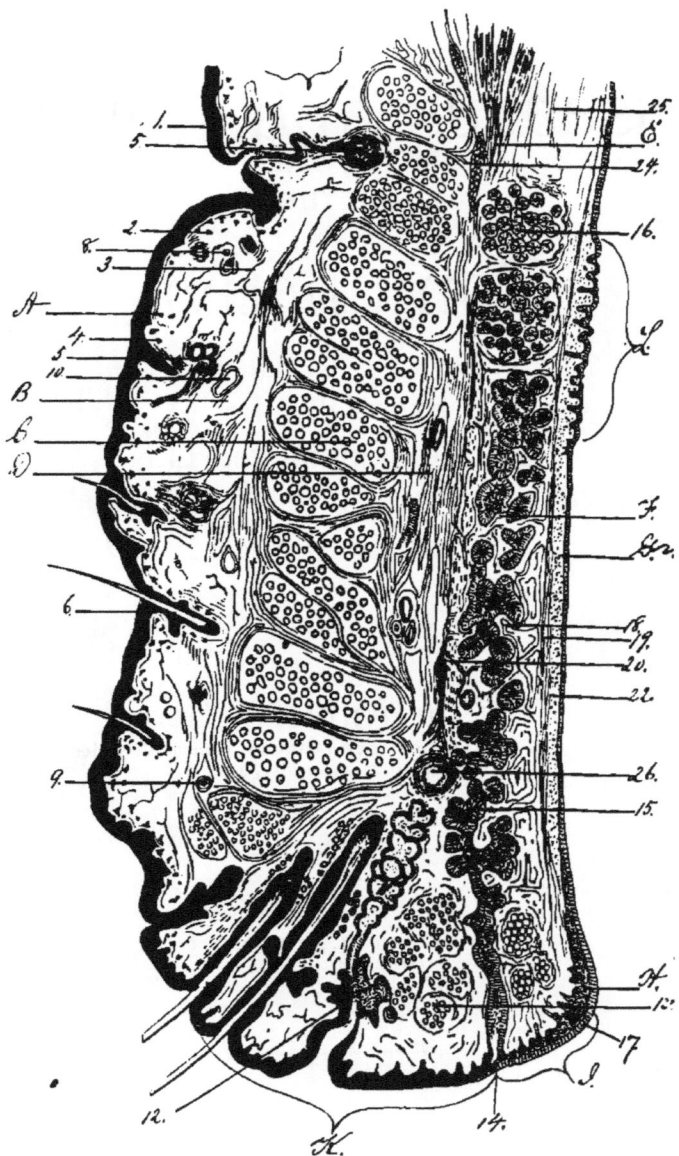

FIGURE 1.
Vertical section through the upper eyelid of an adult man. (Waldeyer)

DESCRIPTION OF FIGURE 1.

A. Skin.
B. Loose connective tissue between the skin and the orbicularis palpebrarum muscle.
C. Orbicularis palpebrarum muscle.
D. Loose connective tissue between the orbicularis palpebrarum muscle and the tarsal cartilage.
E. Insertion of the levator palpebrarum muscle onto the upper edge of the tarsal cartilage.
F. The tarsal cartilage.
G. The conjunctiva of the lid.
H. The epithelium making the cushion at the lower internal angle of the lid.
I. The intermarginal space between the inner edge of the lid and the opening of the Meibomian gland.
K. The ciliary part of the lid from where the eyelashes project and the orifices of the Meibomian ducts.
L. The region of the so-called conjunctival papillæ.

1. Epidermis.
2. Skin.
3. Subcutaneous connective tissue.
4. Pigment cells of the skin.
5. Sweat glands.
6. Hair follicles.
8. Nerve, cross-section.
9. Artery, cross-section.
10. Vein, cross-section.
12. Modified sweat-gland opening into the duct of a sebaceous gland.
13. Muscle of Riolani.
14. Opening of the duct of a Meibomian gland.
15. The Meibomian gland.
16. Posterior tarsal glands under the conjunctiva; evidently belonging to the lachrymal apparatus.
17. Rows of cylinder cells at the beginning of the conjunctiva.
1.. Dense connective tissue of the tarsal cartilage.
19.. The dense connective tissue binding the conjunctiva to the cartilage. The dense connective tissue on the outer surface of the cartilage.
2. Membrana propria of the conjunctiva.
2. Fat cells.
2 5. Loose connective tissue above the upper edge of the cartilage and between the conjunctiva and the levator palpebrarum muscle.
26. Cross-section of one of the larger arteries of the lid.

PREFACE.

The purpose of this little book is to assist practitioners and students of medicine to recognize and treat the diseases and injuries of the conjunctiva. It is not intended that it shall take the place of any of the excellent text-books on the diseases of the eye written by American and English authors, for it is simply a collection of short essays, composed in such a familiar style that those who read them shall not mistake the writer's meaning.

The reason why the author has been prompted to publish the book is, he knows from his experience as a teacher and his observation as a consultant, that the ordinary diseases of the eye are not understood by the majority of physicians, since many of them have neglected the opportunities offered them at their college clinics, and others have not given the eye any attention until compelled to do so, for in general practice the doctor must be prepared for every patient who seeks his help.

Ordinarily, the diseases of the conjunctiva and cornea are not hard to understand, yet that most common of all diseases, granulated lids, is one of the most difficult and important subjects in ophthalmology.

The author, believing that it is possible to simplify the subject "granular ophthalmia," hazards the promise that if the reader will study this book chapter by chapter, beginning at the first and missing none until he has finished the disease chronic blennorrhœa, he will understand what the term "granulated lids" means, and will ever after treat the diseases under that title with more comfort to himself and advantage to his patients.

It is to be admitted that there are some who may not agree with the writer in his ideas of the etiology and pathology of trachoma, chronic blennorrhœa, and follicular conjunctivitis; but, since medicine is not yet an exact science, friendly criticism tends to advance rather than retard its usefulness.

If this little book is kindly received and proves itself of value, it is intended to add to it, in the near future, a similar work on the diseases and injuries of the cornea.

J. H. Thompson, M.D.

Deardorff Building.

TABLE OF CONTENTS.

CHAPTER I.

ANATOMY OF THE CONJUNCTIVA.

The conjunctiva is the mucous membrane which lines the inner surface of the lids and covers the anterior third of the eyeball. When the lids are shut, this membrane forms a closed sac; when they are open, a part of it is exposed to the air. It is possible by careful dissection to remove this sac entirely; then it will be seen that it has one large opening, corresponding to the opening of the lids, and several smaller ones, which give passage to the lachrymal ducts.

That part of the membrane lining the lids is extremely thin, is intimately adherent to the tarsal cartilages; that which covers the eyeball is thin also, loosely attached to the underlying tissue, and is freely movable, excepting the corneal conjunctiva, which, being a part of the cornea itself, cannot be disturbed. The old anatomists taught that the conjunctiva did not cover the cornea, but it will be seen, in the description of the histology of this membrane, that the conjunctiva does not end where the transparent cornea begins.

Between the tarsal and ocular conjunctiva is quite a large extent of membrane, called the retrotarsal folds, forming the superior and inferior cul-de-sacs. There the membrane is somewhat thicker. To the lids it is closely attached, but at the folds it is loose, held in place by fibrous strands from the connective tissue of the orbit. At the internal canthus, external to the car-

uncle, which is also a part of the conjunctiva, is found
a distinct fold of the membrane, of sickle shape, its concave edge towards the cornea, called the plica semi-
lunaris.   This is the remnant of the nictitating membrane of birds.   In man it allows the eyeball to be
turned outwards without hindrance.

It is important for the physician who wishes to treat
the diseases of the eye to familiarize himself with the
normal conjunctiva.

On gently separating the lids, the whole ocular conjunctiva may be seen.   If the eye is slightly cocainized,
it is possible, with a probe, to move the membrane over
the sclera and see how closely it is attached to the edge
of the cornea.   It does not contain many visible blood-
vessels, but they move with the conjunctiva, which dis-
tinguishes them from those which lie upon the sclera and
in the subconjunctival tissues.   In this way, even when
the eye is inflamed, it is easy to tell which vessels belong
to the conjunctiva and which vessels are a part of the
ciliary circulation.   In children the ocular conjunctiva
is very transparent; in adults and those who live in
windy, dusty places the membrane becomes somewhat
opaque, especially that part most exposed to the air; for
which reason we frequently see two triangular areas
of hypertrophied tissue on both sides of the cornea; that
towards the nose being the larger.   However marked
they may be, they never in a healthy eye encroach upon
the cornea.   Close to the nose, at the internal canthus,
is found the caruncle, a small conglomeration of fat
glands and hair follicles.   It belongs to the conjunctiva,
and when the membrane is inflamed, takes part in the
process.   In some eyes the caruncle is more prominent

than in others; it is usually pale red, but on irritation becomes easily inflamed.

The ocular conjunctiva contains many nerves, branches of the fifth, and is plentifully supplied with lymphatics; these, of course, are usually invisible, but sometimes in the conjunctiva of old persons the lymphatic vessels are visible—tortuous, little canals filled with lymph fluid. In young eyes the same phenomenon may be observed, but it is not so common.

When the lids are turned, the palpebral conjunctiva is brought into view. If the inner surface of the lower lid is examined, it will be observed that the mucous membrane is extremely thin and intimately adherent to the tarsal cartilage. It is so transparent that the Meibomian glands are seen arranged in parallel rows, perpendicular to the edge of the lid. Contrary to those of the upper lid, the retrotarsal folds of the lower lid are easily exposed, when it will be observed that the mucous membrane is thicker than on the eyeball and arranged in a fold at the bottom of the lid, more properly in the lower fornix. If it is examined with a lens, nothing more than blood-vessels will be seen; neither follicles nor glands are found in this place, in the healthy eye.

The conjunctiva of the upper lid differs somewhat from that of the lower; it also is thin and adherent to the cartilage, but along the convex edge of the cartilage it is thicker than at the center, varying according to the age of the individual and his occupation. In children the lid is perfectly smooth. In adults, especially those who live in the country, where the eyes are subject to irritation from the wind and

dust, the upper edge of the tarsus is rough and thickened; usually it has a velvety appearance, and through
a magnifying-glass the so-called papillæ may be seen.
It is important to know that this is a healthy condition,
for the doctor may mistake them for granulations. The
reason why the membrane here is rough and thick is a
mechanical one: the cornea presses less against that
part of the lid than at its center.

The color of the normal lid is a delicate pink; but
when the lid is everted, the blood-supply is partly cut off
by compression, then the mucous membrane appears
pale.

It is very important to examine the superior retrotarsal folds.   There the conjunctiva is quite thick, and
forms a large part of the sac.   That part which lies
immediately behind the lid, between the cartilage and
the upper edge of the orbit, is smooth.   If this lid membrane is examined when the superior lid is turned and
pulled up over a spatula, the sharp line of demarkation
between the tarsal and lid conjunctiva will be seen.

The superior cul-de-sac is formed of mucous membrane which covers the connective tissue of the orbit.   It
is plentifully supplied with blood-vessels and lymphatics
and contains a large amount of adenoid tissue.   At the
upper outer edge of the fornix the ducts from the
lachrymal gland open into the sac.   It is not easy to see
the superior retrotarsal folds, for the upper lid must be
turned a second time or the membrane forced into view
by turning the lid and pushing the eyeball into the
socket, while at the same time the globe is rolled down.

Under the outer half of the conjunctiva of the superior fornix and upper lid, above the tarsal cartilage, is

placed the accessory lobule of the lachrymal gland. The secondary gland varies in size: in some it is small; in others it is so large that, when the lid is turned, it is often seen projecting down from above. This anatomical peculiarity should be remembered, for attempts have been made to cut away the gland, mistaking it for a tumor. A like error has been committed regarding the little fold of conjunctiva under the outer canthus, which becomes prominent when the angle of the lids is pulled outwards.

Like all mucous membranes, the conjunctiva is made up of three layers: the membrana propria, the epithelial layer, and the submucous connective tissue. The framework of the membrane is composed of white fibrous connective tissue, with a mixture of elastic fiber. In the tarsal membrane there is little, if any, elastic fiber; in the ocular conjunctiva there is considerable; but at the retrotarsal folds the greatest quantity is found. It is this tissue which gives the conjunctiva its great elasticity. On the surface of the membrane is a distinct basement membrane on which rests the epithelium. Below the membrana propria is the submucous connective tissue, which binds the mucosa to the underlying structures. Over the cartilages there is so little of that tissue that the conjunctiva is practically adherent. At the cul-de-sac the submucous tissue is a continuation of the cellular tissue of the orbit.

Over the eyeball the subconjunctiva is sparing and very loose, but on the surface of the cornea the conjunctiva is condensed to a thin, transparent, homogeneous membrane, called, in honor of its discoverer, Bowman's membrane.* Beween this membrane and the true cornea there is no submucosa, for it is impossible in a healthy eye to remove it without tearing away some of the underlying tissue.

The membrana propria is made up of more than simple white and elastic fibers; it contains numerous connective tissue corpuscles and capillaries. Between all these separate tissues there are irregular, open, and communicating cavities in connection with the lymphatic system. Where the membrane is extremely thin (over the cartilages, for example), the lymph spaces and channels are few. In the ocular conjunctiva they are numerous and large. A fixed connective-tissue corpuscle may contain pigment, or fat; so it is common to find in the mucous membrane over the sclera fat and pigment cells. In the two triangular areas of the conjunctiva, internal and external to the cornea and most exposed to the air, hypertrophied, hyaline-degenerated cells and fat predominate

The lymph spaces contain lymph and lymphatic corpuscles. Some of the spaces are filled with round lymph cells, which can be found throughout the entire conjunctiva, but in some localities the conglomeration of lymph cells is so great that it is called adenoid tissue. This is especially true of the conjunctiva in the upper and lower fornices. The little collections of cells

---

*For certain reasons, which will be explained in the chapter on chronic blennorrhœa and trachoma, it is well to consider Bowman's membrane a part of the conjunctiva. This is a debatable question, so some histologists may not agree with me. But if the reader will accept my opinion in this regard, he will easily understand why the cornea is so frequently attacked in diseases which are purely conjunctival.

are closely related to lymphatic glands, but nowhere in
this mucous membrane are they surrounded by a
capsule or dignified by a separate capillary system;
consequently, there are no lymphatic glands in the
conjunctiva.

Like all mucous membranes, the conjunctiva is covered by two or more layers of epithelium, which are
placed upon a basement membrane separating them
from the membrana propria. The epithelial cells differ
in size and shape according to their function and locality. When the purpose of the cell is to secrete mucus,
it is long and narrow, and its axis perpendicular to the
basement membrane; for which reason such cells are
called columnar cells. When they are to protect the
surface, they are inclined to be flat and arranged in
layers. Beneath these cells are always found some
young epithelial cells, which are small and round. Usually the size and shape of an epithelial cell is modified
by the pressure to which it is subjected. The cells of
the conjunctiva are of one variety, but appear different
in different parts of the membrane. Where the surface
is subjected to pressure, as on the inner surface of the
upper lid, the cell layers are compressed and the cells
nearly flat. On the ocular conjunctiva there are fewer
flat cells, but more round and columnar cells, while on
the surface at the cul-de-sac the cells are chiefly
columnar.

In certain parts the membrane is indentated by folds
and pockets, which are lined with even rows of columnar cells, so that when they are cut across for the
preparation of microscopical sections, they resemble
glands. These so-called glands are scattered all over

the conjunctiva. At the upper border of the tarsal cartilages the membrane is so cut up by grooves and sulci that the surface appears papillary. These papillæ contain vessels and considerable adenoid tissue; but, in a histological sense, they are not papillæ. There are no mucous glands in and no papillæ on the conjunctiva. At the upper edge of the tarsal cartilage in the substance of the upper lid there are a number of little racemose glands, whose ducts open into the cul-de-sac. They are in size and shape very much like Brunner's glands in the intestines. They evidently belong to the lachrymal system; but they are so small that they may be thought to be a part of the mucous membrane. They are under the conjunctiva and are not related to it.

For an account of the nerves, tactile corpuscles, and the development of the so-called goblet cells of the conjunctiva, the reader is referred to the late works on microscopical anatomy.

The conjunctiva passes over the cornea, carrying with it its epithelium, probably some of its lymphatics and nerves, but not the blood-vessels. These stop short at the edge of the transparent tissue. The epithelium is mostly columnar, mixed with round and irregular cells placed *on a basement membrane* and covered by layers of flattened cells. It is true that the cells on the cornea differ considerably in shape and size from those of the surrounding conjunctiva, but in no region of the body is the continuity of tissue more apparent than over the corneo-scleral junction.

When the lids are closed, the walls of the conjunctiva are in apposition; the sac contains no air and very little fluid. The function of the membrane is to permit the lids to move over the eye and the globe to rotate in all directions without friction. The sensitiveness of the cornea is so acute that the slightest roughness is felt. This smoothness of the surface is maintained by the tears and the little mucus which is secreted. If from any cause the surface of the eyeball and cornea dries, and the sensitiveness of the nerves is not benumbed, an irritation is immediately excited, and through it an increased flow of tears. So careful is Nature to keep the cornea moist, that during sleep it is rolled up away from the palpebral slit. Surgeons who have removed the lachrymal glands report that the patients do not suffer from dryness of the eyes, sufficient tears being secreted from the palpebral accessory glands to meet all ordinary purposes. But when the mucous function of the conjunctiva is abolished (in certain forms of chronic blennorrhœa, for instance), the patients complain that the lids seem to stick to the eyeball, especially on waking in the morning.

It is essential for good vision that the surface of the cornea be moist. This is particularly noticeable when a solution of the muriate of cocaine is dropped in the eye. The salt benumbs the nerves both of the cornea and conjunctiva, so that the reflex action on the lachrymal glands and facial nerve nucleus is cut off. The lids do not close every few seconds; then the cornea becomes a little dried. The effect of this on the epithelium is to mar its transparency and, in consequence, the acuteness of vision. The eye is an extremely sensitive organ; for our comfort it is essential that the conjunctiva be healthy.

CHAPTER II.

GENERAL PATHOLOGY.

The majority of the diseases of the conjunctiva are catarrhal or blennorrhœal; so, to treat them successfully, it is necessary to understand the pathology of catarrh and blennorrhœa. This short chapter will be devoted to that subject.

A simple *catarrh* is nothing more than an increased activity of a mucous membrane, which means an abnormal secretion of mucus and serum. The mucus comes from the mucous glands, if the inflamed membrane contains them; from its epithelium, if it does not. In health comparatively few cylinder cells generate or degenerate into goblet cells or suffer mucoid transformation. In disease it is different; many of them become active. There is an active congestion of the membrana propria, and in consequence an over-transudation of blood serum, which, collecting in the membrane and under it, causes an œdema. The overflow passes to the surface, and there, mixing with the mucus, forms the discharge. As the blood serum passes through the membrane it carries along with it some of the lymph cells, a few leucocytes and many of the round cells from the deep epithelial layer. If the inflammation is intense, the serum may contain red blood-corpuscles which have escaped from the capillaries, either through ruptures or by diapedesis. As the process continues, the mucosa becomes filled with leucocytes and newly formed cells.

The epithelial covering suffering considerably; microscopic areas of cell layers are exfoliated, reëstablished, and again thrown off. When the disease disappears, the inflammatory products are absorbed and the epithelium re-formed.

In some forms of catarrhal inflammation a peculiar coagulum forms on the membrane. From some cause which is not understood, the albuminoid and fibrinogenous materials in the transudation coalgulate upon and between the epithelial cells, forming a croupous membrane. It is a yellowish, dirty white deposit of varying thickness and extent, containing many mucus cells and leucocytes imprisoned in a network of fibrin. A true croupous membrane is superficial; it never extends into the membrana propria. For this reason it is presumptive that the exciting cause is either in or on the epithelium. Certain mucous membranes are prone to croupous inflammation, especially that in the larynx and trachea, also the conjunctiva. Croup may accompany acute or subacute catarrh. It is very common in conjunctivitis, for the little white flakes seen in the discharge are of that character. When an acute catarrh loses its intensity and continues indefinitely, it is called chronic catarrh, although there is a difference between subacute and chronic catarrh.

The changes found in the mucous membrane in chronic catarrh are dependent upon the continued hyperaemia. The membrana propria becomes filled with new cells which tend to the development of connective tissue, which ultimately destroys the glandular character of the membrane, if it contains glands, and so alters the normal circulation in the tissues that the

epithelial surface suffers accordingly. The membrane,
at first hyperæmic and thickened, becomes thin, atrophied, and anæmic. These changes are very easily seen
under the microscope. In a transparent membrane,
like the conjunctiva, the atrophy is not apparent, but
it is easy to see the fibrous changes; the membrane becomes opaque, and in some places shrunken.

Blennorrhœa is a suppurative inflammation of a
mucous membrane, the discharge containing a large
proportion of pus—in fact, it is a purulent catarrh.
Like catarrh, there are two kinds of blennorrhœa, acute
and chronic. In acute blennorrhœa the catarrhal condition is intensified; the membrana propria is greatly
thickened because of an exudation of serum and leucocytes. In catarrh it is rare for the albumen and fibrin
to coagulate in the tissues; in blennorrhœa it is the rule.
So dense may be the deposit that the tissues suffer from
pressure anæmia. The filling of the small arterioles and
connective-tissue spaces with white blood-corpuscles
hinders the free circulation of the blood. Thus is established a passive congestion—plenty of blood, but little
nourishment. The result of this may be coagulation
necrosis of certain cell areas of the connective tissue.
Other cells lose their vital tone and succumb to the
attack of micro-organisms or their toxines. In this
way, minute abscesses collect in the tissues and ulcers
form on the surface. In a mucous membrane like the
conjunctiva the swelling will be in proportion to the
looseness of the submucosa. Over the eye the membrane may be one-eighth of an inch thick, and so dense
that when it is cut it will not collapse; at the retrotarsal folds there is nothing to prevent an enormous

swelling of the tissues; on the tarsal cartilage there is a limit.

In blennorrhœa the epithelial coat suffers extensively; all the cells may be exfoliated and the basement membrane destroyed to such an extent that the diseased mucosa is exposed. Sometimes, from certain causes, the fibrin in the discharge coagulates on the membrane; then it is evident that the false membrane on the surface and the deposit in the interior are connected. This is *diphtheria.* Such a false membrane cannot be forcibly removed without tearing away some of the mucosa imprisoned in it. It may melt away and leave the tissue intact; usually, however, it suppurates off, leaving ulcers of greater or less extent. Thus we can understand that an acute blennorrhœa can not last indefinitely, the inflammation will in time destroy the membrane.

Blennorrhœa is always caused by infection. The inflammatory process is the endeavor of Nature to destroy or cast off the invading host of micro-organisms. Some micro-organisms are very active and excite a dreadful combat—the gonococcus, for instance; others are less irritating, but sufficiently offensive to keep up an inflammation more or less intense; such are the streptococci, the staphylococci, etc. Between a gonococcus and a living cell there is no compromise; one of the two must succumb; usually it is the gonococcus. For the time the battle is active, but when it is over, the campaign is finished. For this reason gonorrhœal conjunctivitis rarely becomes chronic.

When a less virulent microbe attacks a mucous surface, it often, in the beginning, excites an acute inflam-

mation.   In time, however, it either loses its virulency,
or the tissues become accustomed to its presence.   Then
the inflammation is less acute and, in consequence,
prolonged.

A blennorrhœa is a purulent inflammation of a
mucous membrane; chronic blennorrhœa is a chronic inflammation of the same kind.   In both the micro-
organisms invade the membrana propria.   In catarrh
the inflammatory new products may be absorbed; in
chronic blennorrhœa the new cells tend to the formation of new growth.   There is, in consequence, a large
increase of adenoid and fibrous tissue.   This over-
growth of adenoid tissue may be diffused over the entire conjunctiva; but in those places where normally
adenoid tissue predominates (in the superior and inferior cul-de-sacs, on the inner surfaces of the lids, over
the internal margin of the tarsal cartilages) the hyperplasia may be very great.   It is these little lymphoid
tumors which form the so-called granulations.   If the
diseased process is stopped, the excessive cell-develop-
ment can be absorbed, as in catarrh and acute blennorrhœa; but in time the cells develop into spindle cells,
connective tissue, fibrous tissue, scar tissue!   The
mucous membrane is more or less destroyed; in consequence, its function is impaired.   Such are the changes
and such the results of chronic blennorrhœa.

CHAPTER III.

EXAMINATION OF THE EYE.

It is necessary, for a proper understanding of the diseases of the conjunctiva, to know how to examine the eye. Ignorance or indifference in this respect may lead to disastrous results. To turn the lids easily and in a moment recognize a disease of the conjunctiva is an accomplishment which can only be acquired by practice. There is no excuse to mistake a catarrh for a foreign body, or to send a patient a long distance to a specialist, who may find a lash sticking out of the punctum lachrymalium. Ordinarily, most of the conjunctival diseases can be recognized at a glance, but the glance must be a searching one. It is important that the patient should be in a good light. One can neither feel nor hear a blennorrhœa; he must see it. The brighter the light, provided it is not direct sunlight, the better; daylight is better than artificial light. The yellow rays in gas or lamp light will mask the true color of the membrane, so much so that an experienced diagnostician may hesitate to give an opinion of a conjunctival disease at night. The examiner should set the patient before the window, if possible; then notice the expression of the eyes and note the position of the lids. Are they swollen? Do they droop? Is there spasm? Are the eyelashes normal in number and position? Is there any moist or dried pus on them? If there is a discharge, is

23

it purulent, mucoid, or principally lachrymal, and does it flow over the cheeks?

He should notice, particularly, the caruncle and the exposed ocular conjunctiva; are they congested, inflamed? Is the disease confined to one eye, or has it attacked both eyes? if so, which the first?

The physician should learn to use a jeweler's glass. It is a great help. Armed with this lens, he should next examine the ciliary border of the lids; there may be scabs at the root of the cilia, he must remove them and see whether they cover ulcers. The next thing is to notice if there are any wild hairs, and see if the puncta lachrymalia are normal in position and in working order. Of course, if the tip of a cilium projects out of the canaliculus and is rubbing against the eye, it will be seen. Before going any further, it is proper to press against the lachrymal sac with the tip of the forefinger and see if any pus wells out from the puncta. If the doctor neglects to do this, he may make a mistake which he will regret.

To see the ocular conjunctiva and cornea, it is necessary to gently separate the lids, which should be done without pressing upon the eyeball. Sometimes, because of spasm and photophobia, this cannot be easily done; a drop or two of a solution of the hydrochlorate of cocaine dropped into the eye will often make the examination bearable; but it must be remembered that cocaine bleaches the mucous membrane.

Following this, one should examine the cornea, looking for foreign bodies on its surface. Are there any ulcers present? Is the cornea clear and transparent?

It is essential to note any abnormality either of the cornea or iris. Is the pupil dilated or contracted?

Now is the time to examine the ocular conjunctiva. Is it inflamed? if so, how much? Is the congestion over the conjunctiva or under it? One must carefully look for ciliary congestion; hunt for foreign bodies; and, if there is a tumor, note its extent and position. The lower lid must be turned down to examine the lower cul-de-sac, and to see the extent and character of any disease that may be there; at the same time to examine the inner surface of the lower lid. Now the upper lid is likewise to be turned to examine the surface carefully. One should look particularly for foreign bodies. Are there any granulations on the lid? Are the Meibomian glands to be distinctly seen, and are there any scars in the mucous membrane, especially near the lid margin?

It is indispensable to learn the difference between granulations of blennorrhœa and trachoma and granulations springing from the bed of a ruptured chalatzion. The examiner should notice the thickness of the lid, and determine whether the tarsal cartilage is hypertrophied or atrophied.

All this may be done quickly, after the student has carefully made a study of only a few diseased eyes. Sometimes it is not so easy to carry out the recommendations referred to above. With children and very nervous persons the examination may be very difficult. It is rare, however, that one is compelled to use a general anæsthetic.

The upper lid is best turned with the fingers. To do this properly, these directions should be followed:

Place the palmar surface of the hand on the side of the head, so that the thumb rests on the upper outer edge of the orbit. Grasp the eyelashes between the thumb and forefinger of the other hand, direct the patient to look down, then pull the lid away from the eye, and with the thumb push the upper part of the lid downwards and inwards; the lid will turn. The lid is not to be turned over the tip of the thumb: it is usually turned from above, not from below. If the lid cannot be everted in this way, turn it over a probe or a thin piece of wood. It is not well to use a lead pencil, for if one is not expert enough to turn it with the fingers, a lead pencil will be awkwardly thick. Older children will usually allow the lids to be turned if they are not frightened by formal preparations and instruments; young children nearly always object. Then it is necessary to be very careful. I usually put the child on its parent's lap and draw it backwards so that its head rests between my knees. By this means, I can hold the head steadily. I then turn the lid over the back of a hairpin. If the child struggles very much and closes the lids spasmodically, it will be necessary to grasp the eyelashes to turn the lid; otherwise the finger simply rolls the lid over. This method of turning the upper lid is recommended especially for infants.

This may seem a trivial thing; it is not. Many eyes have been lost which could have been saved if pressure had not been applied to the eyeball in turning the lid.

When a large child struggles and will not permit the eye to be opened, forcible means are required, especially if it is necessary to see the cornea. Children over six

years of age require an anæsthetic. Younger children
can be examined between the knees or held by assistants; then the lids are separated by elevators.   If
these are not to be had, one may readily make them out
of wire; the back of a hairpin bent over makes a most
excellent elevator.   With these simple instruments the
examination can be made without difficulty.   It is not
advisable to use a spring speculum unless the child is
under an anæsthetic.   Usually when the lids are thus
separated, the eyeball rolls upward.   Then it is necessary to grasp it with forceps and roll it down so that the
cornea comes in view.   It is requisite in these examina-
tions to learn the exact condition of the cornea.   An
infant may be blind when it is brought to the doctor.
If he is careless in his first examination, he may not
recognize the blindness; then in the end he will
be blamed.   This is especially so in ophthalmia
neonatorum.

It is a little difficult to see the retrotarsal folds.
The best way to bring them in view is to turn the upper
lid, direct the patient to look down, then through the
lower lid push the eyeball upwards and inwards with
the thumb of the right hand; the folds will come
forward.   Of course, if there is any disease of the eyeball which makes pressure painful, or the cornea is extensively or deeply ulcerated, it cannot be done.   In the
retrotarsal folds look for foreign bodies and granulations.   If there is a discharge on the membrane, note
whether it is mucus or pus.   In the chapter on the treatment of chronic blennorrhœa it will be shown how important it is to give this part of the conjunctiva the

most careful attention.   An inflexible rule should be: Before the examination and after, *wash the hands!* This should not only be a rule, but a habit.   It may prevent the doctor infecting his patient and may save his own eyes.

CHAPTER IV.

ACUTE CATARRHAL CONJUNCTIVITIS.

Simple acute catarrhal conjunctivitis is an acute inflammation of the conjunctiva, characterized by a more or less intense congestion of that membrane and the exudation of mucus. There is pain, photophobia, and lachrymation. Usually there is œdema of the lids, especially the upper. The first symptom of an attack is an uncomfortable feeling in the eye and the sensation of a foreign body under the lid, which is caused by the enlarged blood-vessels rubbing against the cornea. The sandy feeling usually lasts during the course of the disease, but when the mucus and tears flow, it is, in a measure, relieved. That part of the conjunctiva least exposed to the air is the first attacked; so in the beginning the membrane in the lower cul-de-sac will be most severely inflamed. In a few hours the inflammation will be diffused over the entire conjunctiva, then the caruncle and semilunar fold will become red and swollen. As the ocular conjunctiva becomes involved, the blood-vessels enlarge and increase in number until the eyeball is covered by a network of capillaries. Usually the white sclera shows through the meshes. On careful examination it will be seen that the congestion is confined principally to the conjunctiva. So long as the eye is open and the lids blink every few seconds, the mucus and tears collect about the edge of the lids and are wiped off, but during sleep the mucus dries and glues

the lashes together, so that, on waking, the eye must be
bathed before it can be opened.   The pain may be
moderate or severe.   There is a burning, drawing sensation, which is always worse in the afternoon.   The eye
is so irritable that dust and smoke add greatly to the
discomfort, especially tobacco smoke.   Some people
will not complain much; others, not necessarily nervous
persons, will find it almost impossible to stay in the
light and will have so much pain that the physician may
suspect grave intraocular trouble.

The swelling of the lids varies in degree.   In old
people with relaxed skin the swelling may be so great
that the lids are opened with difficulty and the skin
of the lower lids and cheek looks as if it had been blis-
tered.   This œdematous form of acute conjunctivitis is very common in the aged, and since the conjunctiva may present but little inflammatory evidence
of disease, it may puzzle the doctor to make a correct
diagnosis.

In acute catarrhal conjunctivitis we do not ordinarily see the eyeball very red and covered by large tortuous vessels.   Usually that condition is the result of poulticing, a favorite but dangerous domestic treatment.
When the lids are separated, the sticky mucus will be
diffused over the eye and under the lids, also smeared
over the cornea, which is the only reason for the blur-
ring of the vision.   If this mucus is removed, the cornea
will appear particularly bright and clear in contrast to
the red surroundings; but if its surface is examined
through a lens, it is not unusual to see that in places its
epithelium has been exfoliated, especially at its periphery.   In old people such denuded patches on the

cornea are common. They do not ordinarily go deeper than Bowman's membrane, and heal rapidly. Similar denuded areas are scattered over the conjunctiva, but are not easily seen.

When an eye with a dense pinguecula is inflamed, it presents a peculiar appearance. The pinguecula does not, like the surrounding conjunctiva, become red, so it shows very conspicuously, a yellow-white patch on a red base, at the side of the cornea towards the internal or external canthus. An inflamed pterygium becomes very prominent; an angry, red, fleshy band extending from the caruncle to and over the edge of the cornea.

In acute conjunctivitis the vision is disturbed both by the discharge on the cornea and the distress on accommodation, which is purely reflex; reading cannot be continued any length of time.

This disease is common to all ages, but more particularly in middle life; yet I do not believe that I ever saw a nursing infant suffering from acute catarrhal opthalmia.* Men are more frequently attacked than women. The disease occurs sporadically and in epidemics, particularly in the spring and fall months. It nearly always attacks both eyes, one shortly after the other. Acute catarrhal conjunctivitis may be mistaken for blennorrhœa, iritis, or glaucoma. In blennorrhœa the discharge is purulent. In iritis there is neither mucus nor pus in the discharge; it is lachrymal; the congestion is under the conjunctiva and in the beginning around the cornea; the anterior chamber is clouded, the iris discolored and contracted; the eyeball tender, and the pain more severe at night. If there is any

---

*There is a variety of ophthalmia neonatorum which can properly be named acute catarrhal ophthalmia, but it is a rare disease.

doubt in the differential diagnosis, it can be settled by
the application of atropia: in conjunctivitis the pupil
will dilate fully and rapidly; in iritis it will dilate
slowly, irregularly, or not at all.   To mistake iritis
for conjunctivitis is a fatal error.   In acute inflammatory glaucoma the eye is very red and painful,
the pupil always dilated, the eyeball hard, the anterior
chamber shallow, and the cornea dull. Glaucoma is a
disease of the aged and cannot possibly be mistaken
for conjunctivitis if the physician will be careful.   If
the eyeball is not hard, there is no glaucoma. If there
is a suspicion of glaucoma, the intraocular tension
should be tested before using atropia. In simple acute
iritis the eyeball is apt to be soft.

Cause.—Acute catarrhal conjunctivitis is often
caused by a local irritant, such as dust, smoke, etc. The
most frequent cause, especially in epidemic conjuncti-
tis, is a microbe; although, until the micro-organism is
discovered, it is not unscientific to say that certain forms
of catarrhal ophthalmia are miasmatic contagious. According to our present ideas of inflammation, it may be
correct to say that neither cold nor heat can excite
this disease; but the evidence that local cold may cause
it is so convincing that until it is disproved it is safe to
consider it an etiological factor.   The disease is not
directly contagious—that is, the discharge from one eye
will not create a like inflammation in another. Some
authors believe that it will, and support their opinions
with the fact that there may be several cases in a building at the same time; so there may be two or more
cases of malarial fever in the same house or family,
and it is known that that disease is not contagious.

The *materies morbi* evidently circulates in the atmosphere, for an endemic will be frequently confined to a certain section of a city and among people who are not in any way brought in contact with each other. It may be that the inflammation is the local manifestation of a constitutional disorder, like the subacute conjunctivitis of measles, although it must be admitted that there are no marked constitutional symptoms. The malaise and restlessness are dependent upon the local inflammation. One attack of acute catarrh does not predispose an individual to another. If an eye suffers repeated attacks of acute conjunctivitis, there is in all probability some exciting cause in or about the eye, which may be discovered if sought for.

Prognosis.—The prognosis of acute catarrhal ophthalmia is good, provided the disease is let alone or properly treated. Bad treatment or poulticing may convert a benign trouble into a serious affair. In old people with a tendency to ulceration of the cornea and spasmodic entropion the disease may become intractable, but, as a rule, it will get well. Ordinarily it lasts from three to ten days; it has no tendency to become chronic, and does not naturally leave sequelæ.

Treatment.—The best treatment is rest and the local applications of mild astringents. The patient must be removed from close, dusty quarters to better hygienic surroundings. Bathing the eye with hot water is particularly agreeable and beneficial, but poulticing and continued hot applications are bad; indeed, they are dangerous, and may lead to sloughing of the cornea. If the œdema is not great and the inflammation is severe, cold applications are better; but the attendant

should be careful in using ice-cold compresses in old
people and cachectic individuals.   They lower the
vitality of the tissues, and thus favor ulceration of the
cornea.   As a rule, it is well to let the patient select the
temperature for the water which is agreeable to him,
provided the above warnings are heeded.   The sovereign remedy is the nitrate of silver.   A solution of 5
grains to the ounce of distilled water may be applied to
the inverted lids, and immediately washed off, once a
day.   It is rare that more than three applications are
necessary to effect a cure.   Between these daily treatments the following eye-wash can be used:

R.   Boracic acid.. .. ..1½ drachm.
     Calcined magnesia.. .. .. ½ scruple.
     Water.. .. ..3 ounces.
Mix, filter, and make an eye-wash.

The patient should lie upon a bed or sofa, face up,
so that the pocket at the internal angle of the eye and
nose will hold one-half teaspoonful of the fluid; then
the lids are separated and the wash allowed to run into
the eye.   By lifting the upper lid from the eyeball and
rolling the eye around, the entire conjunctival sac can
be washed out.   This preparation is very soothing; it is
a slight astringent and antiseptic.   It alone will cure
simple acute catarrh.   When it is not convenient to use
the nitrate of silver, any one of the mild astringents will
do.   The acetate or sulphate of zinc, one grain to the
ounce of water, is very good.   Astringents of that
strength may be dropped into the eye three times a day.
It is advisable not to use the salts of lead in eye-drops,
for there is danger, if the substance of the cornea is exposed, of an indelible white deposit of the carbonate of

lead. During the preparation of this article I saw an eye totally ruined by a dense white deposit of the carbonate of lead in the cornea immediately over the pupil. It had been a case of corneal ulcer treated for conjunctivitis with a collyrium of the acetate of lead. Even if the epithelium of the cornea is exfoliated, there is danger of such a deposit forming on Bowman's membrane. This salt of lead, therefore, in a collyrium is not safe, unless the physician who uses it is an expert. A wash of the dilute subacetate of lead (without opium) is a very nice cooling application to the hot, inflamed eyelids of acute conjunctivitis.

It is unfortunate that the acetate of lead behaves in this way, for all the mineral astringents it is the best and the least irritating. Alum is an excellent astringent, 4 to 6 grains to an ounce of water.

A great many physicians order distilled water for the menstruum of a collyrium, which is a mistake. Pure distilled water has an injurious effect on epithelial cells; consequently plain filtered water is better. Another mistake commonly made is the addition of the sulphate of morphine. Morphine tends to irritate rather than soothe a mucous surface. Whenever it is proposed to stop an eye pain with opium or its derivatives, they are better given by the mouth or hypodermatically. Cocaine will relieve pain but for a few minutes, when it must be again given. Unfortunately, this medicine paralyzes the walls of the blood-vessels. Thus it not only aids the congestion, but antagonizes the mild astringents so useful in the disease. My experience is that cold or hot water will relieve the pain of acute conjunctivitis. One of the best local remedies for pain in

the eye, especially if the cornea is affected, is the sulphate of atropia. Unfortunately, the drug causes
paralysis of the accommodation, which does not disappear for some days after it is stopped. Some authorities believe that atropia is dangerous, for it tends to
elevate the intraocular tension in old subjects. This
may be true, but certainly, glaucoma from that cause is
extremely rare. The spasmodic entropion—turning in
of the ciliary border of the lower lid—in old people suffering from acute conjunctivitis can be relieved by hot
applications or painting the skin of the lid with collodion. A simple compress below the lid would be good
if the retention bandage did not prevent drainage.
This condition only lasts a few days during the acute
stage, and will usually disappear as the eye improves.
The sticking together of the lids can be prevented by
smearing the lashes with vaseline on retiring. Under
no circumstances should attempts be made to reduce
the swelling by the application of absorbants, tincture
of iodine, etc. They will irritate and do more harm
than good. If the œdema is so great that the lids can
not be opened—a very extraordinary occurrence in simple acute catarrhal ophthalmia—it can be quickly relieved by multiple puncture, a Graefe cataract knife being the best instrument. There is no danger of this
disease becoming chronic. When the inflammation disappears, the astringent collyria can be stopped, but it
is well to continue for a few days the boracic acid wash.

CHAPTER V.

SUBACUTE CATARRHAL CONJUNCTIVITIS.

Under this heading will be considered certain special
forms of catarrhal ophthalmia, which, in an etiological
sense, cannot be ranked with the disease, simple acute
catarrhal conjunctivitis. They are all subacute catarrhs, non-contagious; some are relapsing and others
have a tendency to become chronic. Chief among these is

SIMPLE CROUPOUS CONJUNCTIVITIS,

a non-contagious, subacute inflammation of the conjunctiva, characterized by the formation on the surface of the mucosa of a croupous membrane. The
disease is more common than is usually supposed,
for a false membrane often forms on the inner surface of the lids in simple ophthalmia in children.
The inflammatory symptoms are not severe. There
may be some swelling of the lids and congestion of
the eyeball. The discharge is not excessive, although
it will glue the lids together at night; there is usually
some photophobia; not much pain. The disease comes
on suddenly and attacks both eyes. On turning down
the lower lid, the membrane in the cul-de-sac will be
found inflamed and swollen; on it long, narrow patches
of yellow-white deposit. Sometimes it is seen on the
ocular conjunctiva, but the most favorite locality is
the mucous surface of the upper lids. This false membrane is quite adherent; it can be removed by rubbing

with cotton and is apt to leave a bleeding spot. It is in all respects a croupous membrane; however often it may be removed, until the disease is well it will return. The amount of false membrane in the eye may be limited or excessive. Sometimes the entire conjunctiva is covered. It can only be mistaken for diphtheria. In diphtheria the inflammation is very severe, the lids much swollen and hard, the eye painful, and the discharge serous. In croup it is easy to turn the lids; in diphtheria it is difficult, often impossible. The false membrane in diphtheria is thick, on an angry, inflamed base; it cannot be rubbed off, and when it is torn away by forceps, it leaves a bleeding surface. In diphtheria the cornea is apt to be attacked; in croup never. In one there are no acute constitutional symptoms, in the other the fever may be high and the pulse rapid. A bacterial examination will make the diagnosis certain.

Cause.—In determining the cause of this disease, it is essential to know whether it is a simple conjunctivitis with a false membrane, or a true croupous inflammation. At present it is not known. Sometimes it appears to be excited by a special germ; then again it has the characteristics of a local expression of a constitutional disease. At any rate, the disease is most common among poor, ill-nourished children living in damp, foul, crowded tenements. Until the bacteriologist solves the question, it is reasonable to believe that the cause is both in the conjunctiva and the blood; there being a special tendency in some individuals to develop croupous deposits on all inflamed mucous surfaces.

Prognosis.—Croupous conjunctivitis, unlike diphtheritic conjunctivitis, will get well and not injure the eye, excepting in some extraordinary cases like the one reported in Chapter XV. There is always some danger of symblepharon, but that is remote. Although there have been reported cases which lasted for weeks, usually the disease is over in a few days.

Treatment.—The treatment should be constitutional and local, good food, fresh air, etc. In some cases the syrup of the iodide of iron and cod-liver oil are necessary. When there is a false membrane on the conjunctiva, it is not advisable to use local astringents; they will do harm. All that is necessary to use in the eye is the boracic acid wash or a mild solution of the bichloride of mercury in salt water, 1 to 4000; 30 grains of salt to a pint of water makes a good menstruum for the bichloride. In very bad cases care must be taken that the conjunctival surfaces do not adhere after the membrane comes away. It is best not to forcibly remove this membrane, or to try to dissolve it by lime juice, papoid, etc.; as long as it is croup it will do no harm. This is a relapsing disease; consequently when the eye is well, the patient should continue for a time the internal treatment and should enjoy the benefits of hygienic surroundings.

CONJUNCTIVITIS PUSTULOSA.

A subacute catarrhal conjunctivitis in which the disease attacks principally the ocular conjunctiva, the mucosa of the lids being not particularly inflamed. The characteristic lesion is a small, shallow ulcer on the conjunctiva, situated from one-eighth to one-fourth of an inch from the edge of the cornea, usually on the temporal side of the eye. The ulcer is on a broad, elevated base, and is, as a rule, covered by the eyelids when they are naturally open. When the diffused inflammation is severe, the ulcer is not prominent; but when the disease is confined to a limited area, the lesion is very noticeable.

Conjunctivitis pustulosa is a misnomer, for at no time is there a pustule. The ulcer does not start from a ruptured bleb, but begins by the falling off of the epithelium from the summit of a wheal. The characteristics of the ulceration are best seen through a lens, when it will be found that its walls are sharp, its floor flat and covered by a faint light gray deposit. The symptoms are much like acute catarrhal conjunctivitis, but less severe. There is a burning pain in the eye, located at the place of the ulcer. The lachrymation may be excessive; as a rule, there is not much mucus discharged. It is rare to find more than one ulcer at a time, the first disappearing before a second appears. This is a relapsing disease; it attacks chiefly young persons, and lasts from five to seven days. It is not dangerous. It must be differentiated from pinguecula, phlyctenular ophthalmia, and especially episcleritis. In the last disease the swelling is in the episcleral tissues, usually very near the cornea, and is never ulcerated. In episcleritis the disease spot is pink and the color deep in the tissue; in conjunctivitis pustulosa it is red, superficial. One is a chronic disease, the other (conjunctivitis pustulosa) comes and goes in a few days. Conjunctivitis pustulosa and phlyctenular ophthalmia are somewhat alike. The differential diagnosis will be considered in the description of the latter disease.

All the circumstances connected with conjunctivitis pustulosa suggest a microbe origin, yet *we do not know.*

The treatment is simple. The boracic acid or bichloride wash is the only local application necessary. Astringents are harmful. Sometimes the healing will be hastened if the ulcer is cauterized or stimulated by touching it with a mild solution of the nitrate of silver; dusting a little calomel into the ulcer is good. If the pain is severe, especially at night, atropia is the best sedative. It not only soothes, but quiets the reflex irritation in the eye itself. Of course, it is essential for comfort to protect the eyes by colored glasses. If the attacks are frequent, there is some local cause; then it is necessary to test the refraction, and, if any error, however slight, is discovered, suitable glasses should be prescribed.

SPRING CATARRH.

The profession was first definitely informed of this peculiar disease by Von Arlt, in 1846. Since then it has been extensively discussed by the German school of ophthalmology, but by the English and Americans little has been said of it. It is strange, for in this great Mississippi valley it is by no means a rare disease. Every year I see many cases. I shall describe the disease as I have found it in the West. It comes under the head of subacute catarrh, for it is not a very acute inflammation of the conjunctiva, nor is it a chronic affection, since, when the eyes get well, all traces of it disappear, although the patient may suffer repeated attacks for years.

In the early spring-time, which in this climate anticipates summer but a few days, some children and young persons will come to the physician with sore eyes; many of them will have simple acute catarrhal ophthalmia, a few the spring catarrh. The eyes are congested, irritable, and watery. The lids are not swollen, but the lashes may be covered with dried mucus and Meibomian secretion. When the patient looks up, the examiner will see distinctly that there is an inflammation of the ocular conjunctiva, particularly around the cornea, for at that place the membrane is slightly swollen and has a tendency to chemosis. At the exact edge of the

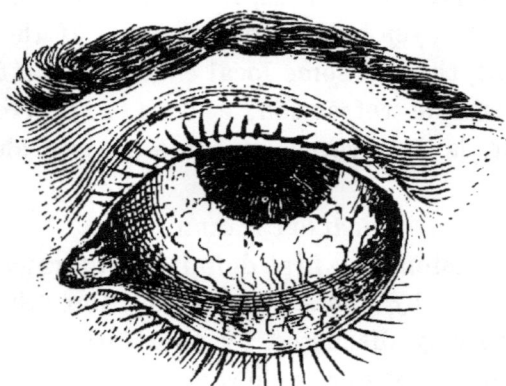

FIGURE 2.

Spring catarrh, showing the irregular thickening of the conjunctiva around the cornea.

cornea *and all around it* will be found little bead-like tumors, some confluent, others scattered; they are waxy red, and, if examined with a glass, will be seen to be in the limbus of the conjunctiva. The cornea immediately adjoining them is clouded, which is very superficial and evidently in the epithelium. The little tumors are caused by an infiltration in the stroma of the

conjunctiva and an active hyperplasia of the superin-
cumbent epithelium.   They are not always small; some
of them may be quite large, one-eighth of an inch or
more across.   At the edge of the cornea they are
sharply raised, but gradually fall off to the level of the
surrounding conjunctiva.   They do not have coursing
towards them large parallel blood-vessels as in phylc-
tenular ophthalmia, but they are covered by a fine capillary network.   The conjunctiva bulbi is distinctly
œdematous and slightly opaque.   In the lower fornix
the membrane is not especially inflamed, but on the
inner surface of the lids it is red, swollen, and rough,
the so-called papillæ over the edge of the cartilages being distinct.   One of the characteristic, I may say diagnostic, signs, which is seen in no other disease of the eye,
is a milky appearance of the conjunctiva, especially in
the lower cul-de-sac and on the inner surface of the lids.
It looks as if a red surface were washed over with a faint
white fluid.   This remarkable appearance is present
in many cases, in others it is absent.   The disease always
attacks both eyes simultaneously.   The patients complain of the light, and some of them of an intolerable
itching of the lids, it being almost impossible to avoid
scratching them.   The eyes are irritable during the day,
especially in the sunlight, but at night or on dark days
they are not so bad.   Studying and close work are annoying, but if the eyes are not taxed they are comparatively comfortable, barring the itching which comes on
in spells.   The disease attacks children and young persons, not infants, and rarely adults.   It comes in the
spring, and often lasts through the summer.   Some patients will be attacked every year, but it has been no-

ticed that as the children grow older the attacks become less frequent and less severe.

The cause of the disease is unknown. It is in all probability not constitutional, for the most healthy children are as liable as the poor and weak. I am inclined to believe that it is the bright sunlight and the warm atmosphere, for unless the eyes are protected from the hot and bright rays of the sun, or the days are cloudy, the disease will not moderate.

The best treatment is a warm boracic acid wash; atropia is very soothing. The usefulness of astringents is doubtful. The nitrate of silver solution, 0.5 per cent, applied to the lids, will sometimes act wonderfully, then again it may do harm. I am in the habit of trying one mild remedy, then another, until I find something that will do good. At bedtime the edges of the lids should be smeared with an ointment of the yellow oxide of mercury, one grain to the drachm of vaseline. . Blue glasses should be worn on bright, hot days. By these means one may cure the disease or moderate its intensity. Usually, in spite of all that can be done, it comes and goes during the summer, to disappear of its own accord in the fall.

CONJUNCTIVITIS OF MEASLES.

All persons suffering from acute, infectious diseases, especially the exanthemata, are liable to inflammation of the eyes. The trouble may be within the eye, in the cornea, or on the conjunctiva. The disease which interests us particularly is the conjunctivitis of measles, the prototype of subacute catarrhal ophthalmia.

This inflammation is as essential to the history of

measles as the eruption, and is always present in a more or less degree. It comes with the dermatitis and is a part of the irritation of the entire respiratory mucous tract. For a long time it was thought it was thought the catarrh extended from the nose to the eyes, but it is believed now that it is excited in the mucosa of the eyes by the *materies morbi* circulating in the blood. It is, therefore, a constitutional disease.

The inflammation in the conjunctiva is a simple catarrh, characterized by some swelling of the lids, congestion of the entire conjunctiva, severe lachrymation, and the exudation of mucus. The eyes are very irritable. They do not pain, as a rule, unless the patient is in the bright light; for which reason the sufferer should always be confined to a moderately dark chamber. It comes on suddenly and tends to disappear in a few days. Unfortunately, however, it is liable to leave behind some slight conjunctivitis, *which may not disappear for months.*

It is not often that the eyes require any special treatment. But should they be unusually irritable and painful, with spasm of the lids, the cornea must be carefully examined. A slight keratitis or a tiny ulcer may be discovered. Then, of course, atropia is indicated. But under no circumstances should any astringents other than the boracic acid wash be used.

CHAPTER VI.

CHRONIC CATARRHAL CONJUNCTIVITIS.

The term chronic catarrh expresses better than any other the diseases about to be considered. In a pathological sense, chronic inflammation means a more or less determined disease, characterized by the formation of a new connective tissue. In ophthamology this is not exactly true, for simple conjunctivitis may last a long time, then disappear, leaving the mucosa absolutely healthy; at other times permanent changes are established; but whether the mucous membrane is damaged or not depends upon the character of the disease and its cause.

In very few organs can a simple chronic inflammation last indefinitely without exciting or inviting some secondary disturbance, which in the end will overshadow it in gravity; for example, chronic catarrh of the bladder, secondary pyelitis; endocervicitis, cancer; in the eye, catarrh, then blepharitis, which by interfering with the drainage of the tears completes a vicious circle. For these reasons a description of a simple chronic catarrhal conjunctivitis may be tedious and difficult, unless one limits his remarks to the original complaint and ignores the secondary diseases, which he cannot always do.

There is a great difference between an irritable conjunctiva and an inflamed one. An individual may awake in the morning and find a little white discharge collected in the internal canthus. Beyond the fact that his eyes look a little dulled, he is not conscious of any trouble. This condition may last a few hours and then disappear until he again subjects his eyes to some irritating matter, usually bad, smoky air. If, during these attacks, the inner surface of the lower lid and the mucous membrane in the inferior fornix are examined, they will be found slightly inflamed. There may be a trace of mucus in the cul-de-sac, but not enough to smear the cornea. It is evident that if the cause is continued, the result will remain, it being the simpler form of chronic catarrh. It is presumptive that such a person has tender eyes, for dust and smoke do not affect the majority of people in that manner. Tobacco smoke is particularly irritable. Some men work on books and smoke at the same time. The heat and fumes from the cigar or cigarette irritate the eyes; a slight conjunctivitis is set up, which may be unnoticed, or it distresses, through sympathy, the accommodation. Very often the sufferer seeks relief in glasses, which, if they are unsuitable, add to the discomfort.

People who work in dusty places, furnace attendants, farmers, and cattlemen have more or less catarrh of the eyes. This trouble is not annoying to them, for they do not read much by artificial light. The disease is very common on the plains, where is is rare to see native adults with clear, transparent conjunctivæ. In adults chronic cartarrhal conjunctivitis does not follow acute inflammation; with children it is different, for following measles it is not uncommon, and many times we are justly suspicious that the foundation for the disease was laid during an exanthematous fever.

That eye-strain can cause continued congestion of the conjunctiva is acknowledged. This is frequently observed among young subjects who are not suffering from great errors of the refraction or accommodation. At the present time there are so many opportunities to get correct glasses that few people fail to seek relief. If the asthenopia is at all distressing, astigmatism is the most frequent anomaly. It is surprising what relief can be got from cylinders of low degrees and how quickly all signs of conjunctivitis will disappear if the proper glasses are worn. The profession was a long time coming to this conclusion, but now that it is an acknowledged fact, there is a tendency to forget that there are other causes for catarrh of the conjunctiva which spectacles cannot remove.

When an irritation like any of the above is continued a length of time, the conjunctiva becomes decidedly inflamed, but the redness will be limited to that part of the membrane least exposed to the air—on the inner surfaces of the lids and on the lower fornix. It is not usual for the eyeball to be inflamed unless the eye is rubbed or the lids disturbed. The conjunctiva at the extreme margin of the lids is inflamed and slightly swollen, which gives a peculiar appearance to the eye, characteristic of chronic conjunctivitis—viz., a red band along the mucous edge of the lid. Ordinarily there is little or no discharge in the sac, but when the eye is disturbed, the tears collect more freely than usual. On turning down the lower lid the pathological changes so characteristic of chronic catarrh are apparent. The mucous membrane is not only thickened, but may be so opaque that the Meibomian glands cannot be seen

It is this condition of the conjunctiva which gives the sclera a slightly yellow amber color. As said before, there is always a tendency in chronic conjunctivitis for the papillæ (?) at the edge of the upper cartilages to enlarge, but they never become distinctly condylomatous, as in blennorrhœa, nor do they appear scattered over the conjunctiva at the center of the lids. The lids may look a little rough; as a rule, they are smooth.

The subjective symptoms are the sandy feeling, burning and irritation of the eyes whenever the patient is in wind, bright sunlight, or artificial light. Many complain that on waking in the morning the eyelids feel dry. All find that close work, like reading, writing, etc., is particularly distressing.

Chronic catarrh of the eyes in children usually takes the form of follicular conjunctivitis, one of the most interesting diseases, which for a long time was, and even now is by some, thought to be related to trachoma.

FOLLICULAR CONJUNCTIVITIS.

In youth there is a tendency to the development of lymph tissue in a mucous membrane when it is irritated. It makes little difference what the irritant is, the consequent congestion tends to the accumulation and growth of adenoid deposits. Consequently, in chronic conjunctivitis in childhood the conjunctiva is often studded with little sago-like bodies, scattered through the stroma of the membrane. The favorite place for them is the lower fornix, where they are arranged in rows parallel to the retrotarsal folds. Under the lens they look like little jelly deposits. They may be discrete or confluent. In bad cases the entire conjunctiva is covered by them,

—4—

but on the inner surface of the lids, where the conjunctiva is thin, they appear like minute blebs. They will
be found in the superior cul-de-sac if they exist in the
lower. The eye is usually a little congested, but when
the lids are turned to examine them, the congestion becomes marked. At other times, on simply looking at
the eyes, not touching them, one would not suspect
that there was anything the matter. Sometimes the
eyes are watery and there may be a trace of mucus in
the corners, but on waking in the morning the lids are
stuck together. The subjective symptoms are the same
as in the chronic catarrh: irritable eyes, which are easily
fatigued. As said above, it makes no difference what
the irritant is, the so-called follicles will appear; often
it is dust, bad air, and smoke; other times it is a septic
microbe. *If there is a chronic blennorrhoea in a child's
eye, the follicles will certainly grow.* This I believe to
be of great importance, for it assists materially to a
better undersanding of a disease not at all uncommon
in this section of the United States—viz., trachoma. A
very frequent cause of follicular conjunctivitis is the
long use of atropia and eserine, especially the latter.
After either of these medicines has been used a certain
time, some eyes become irritable and a slight conjunctivitis arises, which is apt to be follicular. This is not
in any way related to acute local atropia poisoning, to
which some people are liable.

There is a form of catarrhal conjunctivitis which it
is convenient to call septic, for it is caused by a microbe

or its toxines. The germ or poison acts like a specific irritant and excites a subacute, non-purulent conjunctivitis. The disease would have been placed under that heading, Subacute Catarrh, if it were not chronic. It is seen as one of the forms of ophthalmia neonatorum and in disease of the lachrymal sac.

Whenever there is a constriction of the lachrymal canal the tears will accumulate in the sac. Then the microbes and foreign matter washed off the eye collect in the distended sac, where they excite a catarrh or a blennorrhœa. In this place they are nourished, and multiply, and become a medium of infection to the conjunctiva. A vicious circle is completed. This condition may last a long time, but in the end the dacryocystitis becomes purulent. The pus which wells up from the punctum when the sac is pressed upon is extremely poisonous, but it will not generate blennorrhœal conjunctivitis. The most damage it can do the conjunctiva is to inflame it. The poison acts more severely on the cornea, for if that tissue is inoculated by it, it will be destroyed. The majority of cases of abscess of the cornea are from that cause. However severely the conjunctiva may be inflamed, the conjunctival disease will disappear as soon as the sac is opened and drained. The purulent discharge simply irritates the mucosa. These remarks do not apply to those cases of conjunctivitis which are secondary to corneal abscess, they refer alone to the conjunctivitis dependent upon the dacryocystitis. The catarrh of the newborn will be considered in the chapter on ophthalmia neonatorum.

Blepharitis ciliaris pustulosa sometimes follows chronic catarrh; frequently it causes it. The disease at the edge of the lids, particularly the lower, not only destroys the hair bulbs, but causes contraction of the skin to such an extent that the internal margin of the lid and the punctum are turned away from the eyeball—ectropion; the tears then collect in the eye. These, together with the reflected irritation from the diseased lids, excite a catarrh, which will continue so long as the original trouble lasts. That is a serious condition, for when the blepharitis has deformed the lid, it can only be relieved by surgical means, which, at best, are unsatisfactory.

Ulceration of the cornea sometimes happens in acute conjunctivitis; it may also complicate simple subacute catarrhal ophthalmia. The lesions are apt to be long, shallow ulcers in the cornea, near its edge, and not very prominent; so, if the examiner is careless, he may overlook them. They are very easily discovered if the physician uses a jeweler's glass, when it will be noticed that the cornea adjoining them is clouded.

Another kind of ulcer, common in this disease, is irregular in outline, but superficial. The lesion is started by a falling off of the corneal epithelium in persons of low vitality suffering from chronic conjunctivitis; for which reason it is unwise to use cold applications in the treatment of eye catarrhs in the aged. The little superficial corneal ulcers or excoriations are not dangerous, provided there is no disease of the lachrymal sac. If they are the result of chronic conjunctivitis from that cause, the eye is in great danger, for through them the septic material can reach the stroma of the cornea and destroy it.

Treatment.—Before beginning active treatment one should discover, if possible, the cause, which should be removed. The eyes must be protected from all sorts of irritation. It is not a bad plan to test carefully the refraction. Any anomaly, however slight, must be corrected. Very low degrees of astigmatism with axes oblique or against the rule* require correction. The same regarding the phorias.† The best local application for chronic catarrh is the nitrate of silver; a solution 3—5 grains to the ounce of water may be applied to the inner surface of the lids once a day. The medicine should be washed off after each application and not permitted to touch the cornea. The boracic acid wash can be used once or twice between the daily treatments.

Follicular conjunctivitis should be treated on the same principles. As the catarrh improves the follicles will disappear. Children must be removed from all deleterious environments. With them it is not necessary to be so particular regarding the refraction, for

---

*Although the human eye is a wonderfully constructed organ, and for the purposes for which it is intended could not be improved upon, yet, in an optical sense, it is not perfect, for the curved surfaces of the cornea and lens are not accurate. Consequently, a beam of parallel rays of light cannot be exactly focused on the retina. The error is usually such that in the vertical meridian of the eye the refraction is greater than in the horizontal. Therefore, nearly all men are astigmatic in a more or less degree, usually from 0.25—0.5 dioptres. Because such astigmatism can be corrected by a minus cylinder lens axis 180° or a plus cylinder lens axis 90°, and because this is usually the case, oculists say such astigmatism is according to the rule: minus astigmatism, vertical 90°; plus astigmatism, horizontal 180°. If, however, the meridian of greatest refraction is horizontal, or the meridian of least refraction is vertical, the astigmatism is contrary or *against the rule.* Astigmatism of low degree, according to the rule, does not usually cause asthenopia. But when it is against the rule, it is often very annoying, and should be corrected by glasses.

†*Phorias,* a term used to designate the different varieties of insufficiency of the recti or oblique muscles of the eyes. See Tiffany's "Anomalies of Refraction and Accommodation of the Eye," 1896, page 220.

the usefulness of mild cylinder glasses in infants is
doubtful, and little boys and girls do not usually require
spectacles. The mildest astringents are only applicable: 1 grain of the nitrate of silver to the ounce of
water; 1 grain of the acetate or the sulphate of zinc to
the ounce of water;the acetate of lead 2—4 grains to the
ounce; tannic acid 4 grains to the ounce of water and
glycerin mixed; boro-glycerin, made by dissolving
boracic acid in warm glycerin. All these collyria
may be used two or three times a day, excepting the
silver, which can be used but once. It is advisable to
use one remedy for a shorttime,then change to another;
and it is important to remember that after the catarrh
is cured, it will be some time before all the follicles disappear. But, if the irritating applications are continued beyond the necessary time, they will not disappear. A few follicles will do no harm. The sulphate of copper is too severe and powerful for use in
children:some may be tempted to usethe copper crystal,
but they will find that it will do more harm than good.
When the conjunctiva is covered with follicles and the
cul-de-sacs are full of them, they may be removed by
crushing them between the thumb-nails or forceps. In
simple catarrh that operation is rarely necessary. Of
course, if follicular conjunctivitis follows the use of
atropia or eserine, they should be discarded. By add-
ing 1 or 2 grains of the sulphate of zinc to the ounce of
atropia solution, the irritating effect of the mydriatic
may be controlled. It requires long experience for the
doctor to know when atropia is irritating an eye and
when it is not. Eserine, when it irritates, must be
stopped; it is better to do an iridectomy than to con-

tinue the drug under such circumstances. The only treatment for chronic catarrh from disease of the lachrymal sac and canal is to remove the cause by dilating the stricture and cleansing the sac. All chronic diseases are difficult to cure even if curable; they require of the physician skill, and of the sufferer patience.

CHAPTER VII.

BLENNORRHŒAL OPHTHALMIA.

GONORRHŒAL CONJUNCTIVITIS.

The blennorrhœal ophthalmias comprise the most important diseases of the eyes, because of their ˙frequency, their destructive tendencies, and the difficulty of curing them. The prototype of these diseases is *gonorrhoeal conjunctivitis*, which is caused by infecting the conjunctiva with the gonococcus.

The inflammation begins, usually, in one eye like a simple acute catarrh: slight conjunctivitis, some lachrymation, and the well-known sandy feeling; there is some smarting and ocular distress. In a few hours the inflammatory symptoms increase; the lids become œdematous, especially the upper, which swelling enormously projects beyond the lower; the conjunctiva becomes very much inflamed. It is likewise œdematous and swollen. At the edge of the cornea the swelling stops suddenly, so that the conjunctiva is sharply elevated above the level of the cornea—chemosis; the eyeball is very red; there is considerable muco-purulent discharge in the sac and very often the tears are stained with blood. The lids are not hard at this time, so they can be turned, when it will be seen that the membrane over them is fiery red. The pus now commences to flow and collects under the edge of the upper lid; it may run down over the cheek. On the lashes and at the angle of the lids the discharge dries, forming scabs.

There will be considerabe purulent matter in the sac, so that when the lids are pressed upon or separated it wells out, one-half drachm or more. The skin of the lids and adjoining parts is not only swollen, but hot; it looks inflamed. In a few hours there is a change in the appearance of the conjunctiva. The œdema gives way to plastic infiltration; all the inflamed tissue becomes hardened, which makes the turning of the lids difficult and painful. Sometimes there will be found a distinct croupous membrane under the lids, and if the inflamed conjunctiva is much disturbed, it bleeds. The cornea is usually clear, but if the chemosis is very great, it will look small and depressed, and, as a rule, there will be some discharge in the deep corneo-conjunctival angle. Even at this early stage, if the pus is washed off and the surface of the cornea examined, superficial semilunar ulcers may be found near its edge. It may be necessary to push the chemosis aside to see them, when, if they are examined through a lens, they will appear well defined. Such is a picture of ordinary gonorrhœal ophthalmia. Sometimes the inflammatory symptoms are greater, sometimes less. The patient may be restless, have some pain and, perhaps, fever. If the disease is allowed to run its course without treatment, the cornea will necrose. The little ulcers which start at its edge grow larger and expose the corneal stroma to microbic invasion; the entire membrane becomes infiltrated, abscesses form, the eye ruptures, and the cornea sloughs away, allowing the iris and lens to fall forward into the wound. This dreadful accident may happen at any time after the third day. At first the discharge is muco-purulent, then

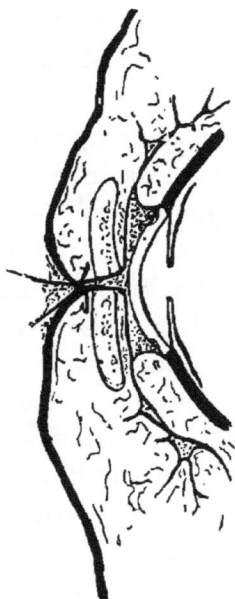

FIGURE 3.

Cross-section of the lids and eyeball in gonorrhœal ophthalmia, to show the swelling of the conjunctiva, the chemosis, the corneal ulcer, and the accumulation of pus.

sanguino-purulent, finally pure pus. About the sixth day the inflammation commences to recede, the swelling of the lids grows less, but the discharge continues freely from ten to fourteen days, when it gradually ceases. The disease lasts about four weeks, and, with rare exceptions, leaves the conjunctiva healthy. So far as the conjunctivitis is concerned, there is nothing more to say; but the lesions to which the cornea is liable deserve further consideration. The cornea may be destroyed by ulceration, abscess, or necrosis. The ulcers usually start at the edge of the cornea under the overhanging conjunctiva; they may begin at any part of the surface. Marginal ulcers are the most frequent;

indeed, it is doubtful if any case of gonorrhœal conjunctivitis escapes them. If the overhanging fold of the
chemosed tissue is not pushed aside in the examination, the physician may not see them, and will be astonished some morning to find the cornea almost surrounded by a ring ulcer. Such ulcers, if not kept clean,
tend to extend towards the center of the cornea and eat
into the anterior chamber. The nutrition of the cornea
is cut off by the constriction of its marginal blood-
vessels under the dense chemosis. The resulting
anæmia destroys the vital energy of the corneal tissue,
and renders it liable to succumb to the destructive action of the discharges. The first symptom of necrosis

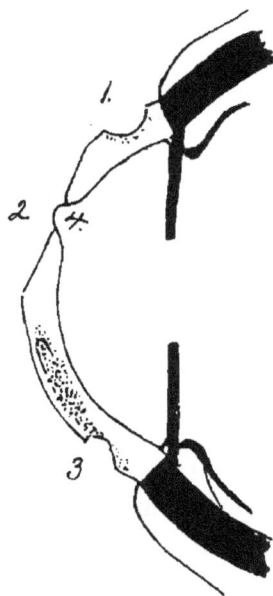

FIGURE 4.

Section of the cornea in acute purulent ophthalmia. 1. Marginal ulcer,
never reaches the edge of the sclera. 2. The glacial ulcer. 4. Shows Descemet's
membrane being pushed through the thinned cornea. 3. Infected ulcer and
abscess of the cornea.

is a deep clouding of the cornea; it becomes white and in a few hours sloughs away. Abscess of the cornea is very common, the purulent process starts at the edge of an ulcer, rapidly extends throughout the surrounding tissue; and thus the cornea is transformed into a layer of pus and rotten stroma. It gives to the intraocular tension and breaks away.

Ulcers which appear during the decline of the disease are very peculiar. They are remarkable in being non-inflammatory, are transparent, shallow, have sloping walls, and look as if parts of the clear cornea had melted away. They have little tendency to perforate, but extend peripherally so that the superficial layers of the cornea may be extensively destroyed. On account of their transparency, they are difficult to see. When they heal, they leave dense cicatrices; but, fortunately, as they are rarely situated in front of the pupil, their opacities do not interfere much with the vision. I have called these apparent ulcers "glacial ulcers," for they look exactly like depressions melted into the surface of a piece of clear ice.

Cause.—The cause of gonorrhœal ophthalmia is direct infection by the gonococcus. It makes little difference where the microbe comes from or how it reaches the conjunctiva, the result is the same. As a rule, the infecting material is carried directly from the genitals to the eye by the fingers, sometimes by towels and washing materials. The urine from gonorrhœal patients can excite the ophthalmia, which is proof that moderate dilution of the pus does not always destroy its infecting properties. About half the eyes are infected by the discharge from a gonorrhœal eye; such pus is as dan-

gerous as that which comes directly from the urethra.
It is presumptive that pus from very acute clap will
cause the most intense ophthalmia and *vice versa.* The
gonococcus seems to lose its virulence when it comes
from a subacute blennorrhœa. Although the discharge
from a chronic urethritis or vaginitis will cause an
ophthalmia, which is apt to be less acute, yet a simple
vaginitis may give the most severe conjunctivitis. Is
there a gonorrhœal antitoxin? Probably; for the
ophthalmia in an individual who is free of clap is apt
to be more severe than in one suffering from acute
urethritis. Physicians and nurses, when they contract
gonorrhœal ophthalmia, suffer dreadfully. One of the
most astonishing things connected with the cause of
the disease is the few who suffer from it in comparison
to the thousands who have gonorrhœa.

Prognosis.—The prognosis is bad; there is great
danger that the eye will be destroyed. The most expert
physicians will lose some cases, the poor or indifferent
ones will lose nearly all. Again, the prognosis depends
very much upon the severity of the inflammation, the age
of the patient, and the treatment. I have never seen a
case of gonorrhœal ophthalmia in which the cornea was
not more or less ulcerated. Young patients stand the
disease better than old ones. The greater the chemosis
the more the danger of destruction of the cornea. The
marginal ulcers are not so malignant as the central lesions, which, if they appear early in the disease, will surely ruin the eye. A clouded cornea is very dangerous, a
milky cornea will slough. Abscess of the cornea makes
the prognosis grave. If the whole or the major part of
the cornea turns yellow, the eye is lost. The glacial ul-

cer is the least dangerous of the corneal lesions. If it appears at the end of the first week, it may destroy much of
the corneal surface and is apt to penetrate; that is, it
weakens the cornea so that the aqueous fluid breaks
through, pushing Descemet's membrane before it. The
glacial ulcer rarely destroys the eye, for when the cornea collapses the melting process stops, and there is
hope that sufficient clear cornea will remain to justify an
operation for an artificial pupil. The longer the lids remain hard the greater the danger. When there is an ery-
sipelatous blush on the skin of the lids and cheeks, it
shows that the conjunctivitis is particularly severe.
Sudden pain in the course of the disease means either
perforation of the cornea or iritis. Ulcers, abscesses,
and necrosis of the cornea, in gonnorrhœal ophthalmia,
progress without much pain.

Treatment.—To treat a case of gonorrhœal ophthalmia with any hope of success requires absolute cleanliness; consequently, if possible, a trained nurse should
be with the patient day and night until he is well. So
much depends upon washing the eye and other little
things which only an expert can do, that, if convenient,
the patient should be sent to the hospital. Home is no
place for these cases. The bed should be small, so the
attendant can reach the patient from both sides. It
should be in a light, airy, cool room, the surroundings
clean, and vessels and materials at hand for the immediate destruction of every rag and piece of cotton
that comes in contact with the disease. The nursing
is really more important than the specific treatment;
therefore considerable space will be given to that
subject.

As a rule, the physician is not called to a case of gonorrhœal ophthalmia until the disease has reached the stage of acute inflammation; consequently, when he sees the case, there is no doubt of the diagnosis. Sometimes he will find both eyes inflamed, often one, which is fortunate, for the second eye will surely be infected by the first unless immediate precautions are taken. The well eye must be hermetically sealed or covered by a watch-glass. When called to a case of ophthalmia in one eye, see if the second is inflamed; if not, proceed as follows:

1. Take a piece of absorbent cotton and wipe the pus off the lids.

2. Clean your own hands carefully with soap and water.

3. Cover the sound eye with a clean rag rolled up and packed carefully under the brow and at the side of the nose.

4. Wipe off thoroughly with moist cotton the face and forehead around the bad eye, starting at the sides and cleaning towards the eye, but don't touch it; now go over the cleansed area with a solution of the bichloride of mercury 1: 2000, but be careful that the fluid does not wet the rag on the good eye.

5. Cover the diseased eye with a big bunch of antiseptic gauze; then wash your hands again, and clean the other side of the face, working from the eye outwards, but be careful not to touch the lids, although the angle at the nose must be carefully cleaned; go over with the bichloride 1:2000, and dry thoroughly.

The eye is now prepared for sealing. Over the closed lids put a thin layer of absorbent cotton, then fill up the depression with little pieces of iodoform gauze.* Cover the whole with a piece of oiled silk and fix the edge to the skin with silk plaster. Cover this with collodion, and be especially careful that the covering sticks tightly to the bridge of the nose. Such a packing will prevent any fluids from the opposite side reaching the eye. The dressing should be removed every third day. If there is no pus on it, it is not necessary to open the eye; so long as it is not diseased, keep the lids shut. Some prefer to shield the eye with a watch-glass. It has an advantage over the pack, since the eye can be seen, is well ventilated, and the patient is not blinded. Wash as advised in the first instance. Take a clean wash-glass and fix it to the brow and nose with silk plaster; cover the plaster and skin with collodion. Whenever the plaster comes loose, remove the glass, clean it, and re-apply it. If this is done in time, disease of the second eye will be prevented. The patient must keep his hands away from his face and be warned of danger.

A great many specialists doubt the usefulness of constitutional treatment for this disease. They may be correct, but it does seem rational to combat the inflammation by such internal remedies in use to control acute diseases elsewhere. We have no specific to rely on, but we have certain drugs which tend to modify the intensity of acute inflammation. 5—6 grains of calomel at night, followed in the morning by a glass of Hunyadi János water, will not only clean out the bowels, but act as a derivative. Veratrum viride to soften the pulse or aconite to relax the skin, are useful. If the

*Do not put iodoform gauze next to the skin of the face in a permanent dressing, unless you know that it will not irritate.

inflammation is very severe, small nauseating doses of tartar emetic continued for 24 hours are advisable. In fact, all constitutional antiphlogistic means at our command should be made to assist the local treatment. *The risk is too great to play with fancy drugs; give the good and reliable ones freely.*

The object of local treatment is to keep the inflammation under control and save the cornea. It is questionable if any application can stop the progress of the disease if it gets a good start, although we can cetainly modify its intensity if we see the eye before the acute stage is reached. If one knows that infecting material has reached the conjunctiva, which sometimes happens to attendants in washing a diseased eye or urethra, he must immediately proceed to remove or destroy the germs. Place the individual on his back and wash out the conjunctival sac with warm salt water, according to the method advised in using the boracic acid wash. Be sure the fluid reaches the upper cul-de-sac; then wash out with a solution of the bichloride of mercury 1:2000. Don't use us it in drops, apply it copiously and thororoughly; then apply ice-cold compresses for an hour; go over the same process again in about two hours. Instead of the bichloride, the nitrate of silver, 8 grains to the ounce of water, may be dropped into the sac. Use 4 or 5 drops and let them run over the eyeball, follow with cold applications to relieve the smarting. When about to use silver, wash with plain water, not salt water; the salt destroys the silver, but adds to the efficacy of the mercury. This solution of silver will cause considerable reaction, which must not be mistaken for the disease. The artificial conjunctivitis should dis-

appear in a few hours.   If a large quantity of pus or
purulent water reaches the eye, there is little hope
that the disease can be aborted.

When the lids are very much swollen, apparently
pressing upon the eyeball, and there is great chemosis,
to avoid sloughing of the cornea, relieve the tension.
Give an anæsthetic; then with a pair of strong scissors
cut the external canthus out to the bone; put the forefinger under the upper lid and raise it from the eyeball;
the so-called external tarsal tendon will be distinctly
felt holding the lid to the bone; with a pair of sharp-
pointed scissors nick the tense tendon until it gives
way, but be careful not to cut the skin.   One blade of
the scissors should go into the sac, the other between
the tendon and the skin.   This will immediately take
all pressure off the eye.   Permit the wound to bleed
freely.   While the patient is under the anæsthetic, test
the chemosis with the finger;if it is hard, scarify it; the
cuts should radiate from the cornea.   Clean out the
sac with a solution of the bichloride of mercury 1—3000,
and keep on the lids continually ice-cold applications.
The eye must be washed with the mercurial solution at
least every two hours, often enough to keep it clean of
pus.   In washing the eye use an eye-dropper, which
can be pushed up under the lid; syringes are bad and
dangerous.   So long as the acute process lasts, nothing
more can be done to protect the cornea.   Some surgeons
advise hot applications in preference to cold, claiming
the swelling goes down quicker and that the heat has a
good influence on the disease.   This may be true.   I
know that cold is good, for it is the bridge over which I
have many times successfully crossed.   As soon as the

lids can be easily turned, but not before, begin the nitrate of silver treatment. Ten grains of the nitrate of silver to the ounce of water should be the strength of the solution; apply it with a camel's-hair brush to the inner surface of the lids, then wash off with plain water, not salt water. The object is to allow a diluted silver solution to reach the eyeball. The silver acts not only as an astringent, but as an antiseptic. All other astringents, fancy compounds, and iodoform are useless. He who sticks to the silver will save the most eyes. These applications should be made twice a day until the discharge ceases, but as the eye improves the strength of the solution may be reduced. The wound at the angle of the lids will heal without any attention. If there are deep ulcers on the cornea, great care should be exercised in turning the lid, for there is danger of perforation if any pressure is applied to the eyeball. We can do nothing for abscess of the cornea, but hope that when the disease disappears sufficient transparent cornea will be left for an iridectomy. I do not know the cause of the glacial ulcer and know no way to stop its progress, unless it be paracentesis. This may be tried, but it is dangerous. The chief object of all treatment is to keep the cornea as clean as possible and prevent pressure on the eyeball. It is a question if the nitrate of silver will shorten the disease many days. A gentleman wearing an artificial eye contracted gonorrhœal conjunctivitis on the blind side. I saw him before the inflammation reached the very acute stage. He was put to bed in a private hospital, given a special nurse, and the good eye covered with a watch-glass, every care being taken to prevent secondary infection. Twice a day I separated the lids with a spring speculum and cleaned out the orbit thoroughly. I then swabbed it with a 10-grain solution of the nitrate of silver. The orbit was, moreover, cleaned out with a solution of the bichloride of mercury 1:3000 every two hours day and night. The discharge was not so plentiful as is usual in gonorrhœal ophthalmia, but the disease lasted one month. This was a case to test the abortive effect of the nitrate of silver. My experience is, that treatment simply controls the inflammation; the disease must run its course.

CHAPTER VIII.

OPHTHALMIA NEONATORUM.

By common consent, all kinds of conjunctivitis, whether purulent or not, which attack children from three to six days old, are called ophthalmia neonatorum. If the term "ophthalmia" means in this sense a purulent disease, it is a misnomer, for diseases of the conjunctiva in the newborn are not always suppurative, Simple catarrhal conjunctivitis can arise in the early days of life.

The usual ophthalmia is an acute purulent conjunctivitis, and has nearly all the characteristics of gonorrhœal conjunctivitis. The inflammation may be as severe as gonorrhœal, but usually it is much milder.

Between 24 and 36 hours after the child is born a slight swelling and congestion of the edges of the lids is observed; there will be a little muco-purulent discharge, which collects at the angle of the lids and on the lashes. Very soon afterwards the inflammation will be established. If it is to be a severe case, the swelling may equal that of acute ophthalmia; commonly it is decided, but not excessive. Then the matter begins to flow freely; it may run down over the cheek, and, because the bridge of the baby's nose is flat, it easily reaches the other eye. Usually both eyes are diseased. If the eye is now examined, the conjunctiva will be seen very much inflamed, but the membrane covering the eyeball will not be so œdematous as in purulent disease in the adult, nor will the chemosis be as prominent. At first there will be some difficulty in turning the upper lid, but in a few hours it can be easily done, because of the swelling of the tissues of the superior retrotarsal folds. Often this swelling resembles granulations, and when the upper lid is turned

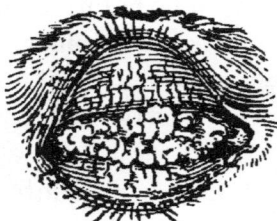

FIGURE 5.

Ophthalmia neonatorum, showing the granulations which sometimes project from the upper cul-de-sac when the lids are turned.

they spring into view, a red, granular, suppurating mass. This condition may prevent the lid closing down on the eye. At other times the swelling is so great that when the child cries the upper lid turns out of itself. The inner surface of the lid is very red, often covered by patches of croupous membrane, and, if it is roughly handled, will bleed.

The cornea is apt to ulcerate, the ulcers starting at any place and very rapidly progressing. The cornea may slough away entirely, which, unfortunately, is a very frequent occurrence; the corneal lesions being exactly like those found in gonorrhœal ophthalmia. Such an inflammation will run from 3 to 6 weeks. In some cases there is not so much swelling of the tissues. The discharge, instead of being thick, yellow pus, is creamy white and profuse. When the lids are turned, the retrotarsal granulations do not come in view; such a condition one would expect in subacute ophthalmia. In the first case the lids are usually closed; in the latter they may be open from time to time. Even in the modified disease, the cornea is in danger. There is another variety of ophthalmia, in which the inflammation is very slight, some irritation, congestion and slight discharge of pus, enough to glue the lids together during sleep and collect about the lashes; the child keeps its eyes open, they are irritable, and there is evidently some photophobia.

The catarrhal ophthalmia begins about the fourth day; the lids are not red nor swollen, but the eyes are slightly inflamed, the conjunctivitis being principally behind the lids; there is some mucous discharge and excessive lachrymation; the eyes look as if the tear-ducts were closed. There is evidently some photophobia, for the child avoids the light. Thus it is seen that ophthalmia neonatorum may be of all grades, from the simple catarrh to the most profound blennorrhœa.

Cause.—Ophthalmia neonatorum is nearly always caused by the conjunctiva being infected by the discharge from the maternal vagina during the passage of the head. There is no reason why the disease cannot be contracted from dirty clothes and fingers. One thing is certain, the *materies morbi* comes from some genital mucous surface. Bright light, dirt, smoke, and soap do not cause it, so the popular opinion that careless nurses are responsible is a cruel mistake. The origin of the disease is often gonorrhœa. This statement is at present in dispute. Because a child's father had gonorrhœa months, or perhaps years, before is no proof that his trouble had any thing to do with his offspring's misfortune. There is strong evidence to the contrary, for I have seen the disease in children of parents who never had gonorrhœa.   When gonorrhœa is the *immediate* cause, there are no doubts, because the inflammation is dreadfully severe and the gonococcus can be found in the discharge.   That simple leucorrhœal pus can cause ophthalmia is undoubtedly true; in fact, there is reason to believe that a purulent discharge from the genitals, whatever be its character, is poisonous to the eye.

Prognosis.—If a case of suppurative ophthalmia runs its course without treatment, the prognosis is very bad; eighty times in a hundred the eyes will be destroyed.   Some may have damaged eyes and some may recover from the disease with good vision.   When an infant receives proper treatment and care, the prognosis is good.   There is little excuse for a physician to lose an eye if he sees the case early and attends to it carefully until it is well.   If the eyes are infected by gonorrhœal pus, the progress is doubtful, but not so bad as the same disease in the adult.   Under the best care the cornea may slough.   Slight ulceration does not endanger the eye very much, for few cases of severe ophthalmia recover without some corneal lesion.   A rapid clouding of the cornea precedes sloughing but a few hours, but that is not apt to happen unless the eye is neglected.   If one eye is diseased, the second rarely escapes.   The configuration of a baby's face and nose makes bandaging impossible, and certainly no one would attempt to fit a watch-glass.   Mild cases require as much attention as severe ones, for it is surprising to see how rapidly the cornea may slough, even though the lids are not swollen.   So long as there is any pus secreted, there is danger. The disease lasts from three to five weeks.

Simple catarrhal ophthalmia neonatorum is not at all dangerous. It is tedious and annoying to physicians; it lasts for days, even weeks.

Prophylaxis.—Within recent years it has been found that it is possible to save children from an attack of ophthalmia, even though the mother has suffered from leucorrhœa up to her lying-in. In all large maternity hospitals the prophylactic method of Credé is a routine practice. It has enormously reduced the percentage of infantile ophthalmia. For this purpose he suggests a most powerful, yet harmless, antiseptic. It is a 2 per cent solution of the nitrate of silver—9—10 grains of the salt to an ounce of distilled water. It should be freshly prepared before use. When the baby is born, wipe its face with a clean, damp cloth, then dry the skin about the eyes. It is well to start the cleaning at the eyes, as suggested in the chapter on gonorrhœal ophthalmia. The eyes are by no means always infected, although poisonous matter may be on the face; so if the physician carelessly washes the face, he may infect the eyes himself. As soon as the child is washed and dressed, separate the lids and drop in two drops of the silver solution, allow it to remain a second or two, then close the lids and wipe off the escaped fluid. One application is sufficient; the eyes recover from the treatment in a few hours. The disease will be prevented in 95 per cent of cases, even if the conjunctiva is infected. If a quantity of gonorrhœal pus has entered the eye, Credé's method may prevent ophthalmia, but I doubt it.

Treatment.—There is no disease of the eye which will respond so certainly to correct treatment as this. But it must be remembered that the eyes require the most careful attention until all traces of the inflammation are gone. It is dangerous to turn over an improving case to the care of the nurse or mother. A very competent oculist was treating a case of ordinary ophthalmia neonatorum: he used the nitrate of silver and had almost cured the child; he then prescribed a wash, and left the city for a few days; when he returned he found the inflammation as bad as at first and both corneas sloughed away. We often hear physicians speak of the virtues of alum water, sulphate of zinc, pyoktanin, etc. They may be good and may cure some cases, but there are others they will not cure. The risk is too great to rely on anything but the nitrate of silver. It is true that keeping the eyes clean by washing them every hour or so is good treatment, but no one should depend on that alone. Whatever be the character or degree of the inflammation, the treatment should be the same.

The best treatment is the local applications of a solution of the nitrate of silver 3—20 grains to the ounce of water. Sometimes it is necessary to make it stronger, and when the granulations are excessive, the mitigated stick* may be used. The condition of the cornea should not modify this treatment whatever. When a physician is called to a case of infantile

---

*ARGENTI NITRAS DILUTUS, *U. S.*—DILUTED NITRATE OF SILVER. *Argentum nitricum fusum mitigatum, Lapis infernalis nitratus.*

Preparation.—Nitrate of silver 1 part; nitrate of potassium 1, 2, or 3 parts. Melt the salts together in a porcelain crucible at as low a temperature as possible, stirring the melted mass well until it flows smoothly. Then cast it in suitable moulds. Keep the product in dark amber-colored vials, protected from light.—*U. S.*

ophthalmia, he must be sure to examine the cornea, for the prognosis should be made at the first visit. If the cornea is badly ulcerated or necrosed, the relatives must be informed; for if the child loses its eyes, they will blame the physician, while they praise the one who stops the inflammation, even if they know the eyes are destroyed. The eyes must be kept scrupulously clean; the matter removed from the lids as soon as it accumulates. The eye is best washed with an ordinary dropper, the lids being separated, and the fluid applied drop by drop. Water will do, but the bichloride solution 1:3000 is better; of course, care must be taken that the fluid does not enter the mouth or run down the nose, for this preparation of mercury is a little strong. It is doubtful if weaker solutions have any antiseptic virtues. If, on turning the lids, a mass of granulations springs forward from behind the upper lid, they should be carefully cauterized by the mitigated stick or a 20-grain solution, but the silver must be immediately neutralized by salt water. The cauterization may be made once a day. It is surprising to see how rapidly such bad cases improve. If there are no granulations, apply to the inverted lids a 10-grain solution of the nitrate of silver, wash off with plain water; all the silver must not be neutralized, a little should reach the eyeball. This application should be made morning and evening; sometimes it is necessary to use a stronger solution. The pyorrhœa should moderate immediately. When the excessive flow stops, the intervals between the treatments may be lengthened, but it is not advisable to use less than a 1 per cent solution until the discharge stops entirely. Even then the case must be watched a few days, for there is danger of a relapse. It is not necessary to examine the cornea at every visit. As soon as the discharge commences to diminish, the cornea will improve, and all ulcerative processes stop. The most encouraging sign is to find that the child opens its eyes, which shows that the swelling is going down, and that the case is on the way to recovery. True gonorrhœal ophthalmia in an infant requires the same treatment as the disease in the adult.   Canthotomy may be necessary to relieve the tension, but one must not wait until the acute stage moderates before commencing the silver applications.   A bleeding conjunctiva is not a contra-indication to this treatment.

It is surprising how rebellious and annoying the simple catarrhal ophthalmia may be.   The best treatment is the nitrate of sliver, 5 grains to the ounce, applied once a day.   During the treatment of opthalmia neonatorum the child must be kept in a clean, well-ventilated, cool room.   So keep the infant away from the stove, and do not let it get heated under a pile of bed-clothes and shawls.   This is one of the most difficult regulations to introduce, for parents and nurses have an idea that the baby must be kept hot or half-smothered.

CHAPTER IX.

LEUCORRHŒAL OPHTHALMIA.

As before stated, there is a strong suspicion that any purulent discharge from the urethra or vagina will excite ophthalmia if it reaches the conjunctiva. Ophthalmia neonatorum is caused in this way, although the contagium may not be related to gonorrhœa. Those who practice in large dispensaries meet cases of conjunctivitis which it is convenient to call leucorrhœal ophthalmia. The conjunctiva is very much inflamed and the eyeball very red; there is some swelling of the lids so that the upper lid droops—partial ptosis. There is no chemosis; the cornea is clear and remains so until about the second week, when superficial keratitis and the development of blood-vessels occur. There is always a muco-purulent discharge and the eye is extremely irritable. The disease usually attacks one eye first, but the second may be infected by the discharge from the first. There is no characteristic symptom, but in every case the tarsal conjunctiva will be found quite rough, deeply congested, and velvety. The disease tends to become chronic.

I have no proof that it is caused by leucorrhœal matter, but every case I have seen was evidently of that character. A little girl four years old was attacked by a severe purulent ophthalmia. She was the child of well-to-do people. She had not been out of the house for several days before the eye inflamed. On

77

inquiring into the cause of the ophthalmia, I found that
the mother was suffering from a profuse chronic, non-
gonorrhœal leucorrhœa.   The father was healthy.

A young woman consulted me for an attack of subacute purulent conjunctivitis; she, too, was suffering
from a non-specific leucorrhœa.   I have seen many
other cases of like character, when it was not prudent
to inquire too strictly for the cause.   The disease differs
from the initial stage of chronic blennorrhœa or granular ophthalmia is one important respect.   It is not
difficult to cure, and, if properly treated, it will not become chronic; yet, if neglected, it may run into a condition which cannot be differentiated from granular
ophthalmia.

The best treatment is the nitrate of silver, a 2 per
cent solution applied to the tarsal conjunctiva once a
day.   This medicine will smart considerably, so it is
well to bathe the eyes afterwards with cold water.   The
mild astringents will do no good, and it is not safe to
rely upon simple antiseptic collyria.   In using the
silver be careful not to let it come in contact with the
cornea.   That tissue does not ordinarily ulcerate, but,
if it is irritated, it will inflame.   Hot eye-baths are
sometimes beneficial, but warm applications and poul-
tices are dangerous.   It is advisable to keep the eye
under the influence of atropia.   It should be protected
by smoked glasses, and the patient must avoid a smoky,
dusty atmosphere.   If the silver is used in the morning,
is not a bad plan to wash out the eye at night with the
bichloride 1:2000.   Should this solution smart severely,
it may be diluted to 1:3000.   It is important to keep up
the treatment until the eye is perfectly well.   As the in-

flammation improves the strength of the silver solution can be diminished, then the boracic acid wash
substituted.

Inflammation of the cornea does not contra-indicate
this plan of treatment, but it should be irritated as little
as possible.

CHAPTER X.

GRANULATED LIDS—TRACHOMA—CHRONIC BLENNORRHŒA.

It is doubtful if there is any subject in ophthalmology more important or interesting than granulated lids, *vel* trachoma, *vel* chronic blennorrhœa. This statement is based on the fact that in this Western country there are more people suffering from chronic sore eyes than any other single disease. It is true more die from consumption than lose their sight from chronic blennorrhœa; but there is not a town of 2,000 inhabitants in Missouri and the adjoining States in which there are not from 20 to 30 persons with some disease of the conjunctiva. In our large cities the percentage is even greater, and one need only visit the dispensaries to find how much more prevalent it is than all other ophthalmic cases. Although chronic disease of the conjunctiva does not add many to the blind list, it makes an enormous number of persons utterly miserable and causes the loss of thousands of dollars by rendering so many incompetent to work. It is the oculist's *bête noire*, ever present in his office, ready to rob him of his comfort, his reputation, his conceit, and his time.

Any one of ordinary experience with the disease must have some idea concerning its cause and treatment. Hundreds have written of granular ophthalmia, yet it is by no means certain that any one has mastered the subject. Instructed by one of the best authorities on the diseases of the conjunctiva (Von Arlt), and closely studying every case it has been my fortune or misfortune to treat, I have also reached some conclusions, which I present for what they are worth, and hope that they may assist some to a better understanding of the subject and materially aid to the relief of many who suffer now and will in the future.

One peculiarity which makes the study of this disease so difficult is the fact that it differs greatly in different parts of the world. A German or an Austrian writer may be an authority in his own land and his book be of little assistance to a practitioner in the Mississippi valley. Few men in London know anything of Egyptian ophthalmia, and it is doubtful if a New Yorker could formulate a plan of treatment to be carried out with any great hope of success in Kansas City. I take it this is one of the reasons why the profession does not agree. Schweiger, in his text-book on the diseases of the eye, says, "The sovereign remedy for acute granular ophthalmia is the sulphate of copper." Evidently this is true in Berlin, but here I find that copper is often very unsatisfactory, and will not cure 10 per cent of the cases. In Vienna I have seen many cases which I shall call simple, pure trachoma; in this Western country I have seen comparatively few. At the American Medical Association I have heard my Eastern confrères discuss the subject, when I have been forced to the conclusion that in the United States there is a variation in type of the disease called trachoma. Therefore I believe it would be a waste of time and a confusing task to quote the many authorities both in this country and abroad. In the pages devoted to this subject

I shall give my own ideas, with the understanding that what I write refers to the disease called granulated lids in this great, western, central valley.

Under the title "Granulated Lids" are three separate and distinct diseases: 1, Trachoma; 2, Chronic Blennorrhœa; 3, Follicular Conjunctivitis. An individual may suffer from any one of them and have what the doctors call granular lids. He may have at the same time any two of them—trachoma and chronic blennorrhœa; chronic blennorrhœa and follicular conjunctivitis; trachoma and follicular conjunctivitis; indeed, the three may be combined in the same person. It is this tendency to mix the diseases which makes the subject so difficult. For convenience, it is best to describe them separately. Follicular conjunctivitis has already been considered; consequently I shall begin the subject "Granulated Lids" with a description of the disease called trachoma.

TRACHOMA.

An infectious disease of the conjunctiva, characterized by the growth in the stroma of the membrane of a number of little round sago-like bodies called trachoma follicles. The nodules are about the size of the head of an ordinary pin; they are colorless, very much like the follicles in common, follicular conjunctivitis, but differ from them in that they are smaller and harder. They may be scattered over the entire conjunctiva, but in those places where the mucous membrane is thick, succulent, and filled with adenoid tissue, they are most numerous. So it is not unusual to find the retrotarsal folds, especially the upper, so thickly covered by them that when the lids are turned they spring into view like a mass of frog's spawn.

In the lower cul-de-sac there are never so many, but in all cases the trachoma bodies will be found deep under the inferior lid, if the examiner will use a magnifying-glass. A very favorite locality for them is the convex edge of the upper tarsal cartilage, where they are usually quite large and distinct. They may be scattered more or less abundantly over the inner surface of the upper lid, but there they differ in appearance according to their depth. On the surface of the membrane, they are distinct, round tumors, so when the finger is passed over the lid there is a decided roughness; but, in the cartilage the neoplasms are small and diffused and appear like little, round, white specks about one-twenty-fifth of an inch in diameter. Such an eruption may be in an eye very little, if any, inflamed; indeed, the conjunctiva can be anæmic. This is what is called simple non-inflammatory trachoma, a disease rarely seen in this part of our country, but common in Europe. In nearly all cases there is a slight conjunctivitis; the eyes are irritable, and there is a little muco-purulent discharge, enough to slightly glue the lids together at night. The trouble may thus insidiously progress for months, when suddenly there is a sharp attack of acute inflammation, and in an hour the entire character of the disease changes.

Acute inflammatory trachoma is simple trachoma plus acute conjunctivitis. Sometimes there is an inflammatory œdema of the conjunctiva and lids, considerable photophobia, especially if the cornea is attacked; the lids are tightly closed, and when they are forcibly opened, a quantity of tears, mixed with mucus, flows out. The entire conjunctiva is inflamed, that covering the eyeball is very red. Because of the swelling of the membrane, the trachoma nodules are not so prominent as in simple trachoma, but they can be easily seen. It appears that the tarsal cartilages are also inflamed, for they are much enlarged, both in length, breadth, and thickness. The condition of the lid will depend upon the stage of the disease. Trachoma may attack the eye as an acute inflammation, when, of course, all that will be seen is an eruption of small nodules on an acutely inflamed conjunctiva. Usually, however, the inflammation attacks an already diseased mucosa, then the neoplasms will be found confluent, deep, in places cicatrized. It is in such cases that the upper tarsal cartilage is hypertrophied, because of the œdema, the trachomatous infiltration, and the thickening of the mucous membrane.

It is very rare that the only trouble in the mucous membrane is the trachoma. On the inner surface of the lids, especially the upper, the conjunctiva is often hypertrophied; at least, there is an increase in the normal adenoid-tissue and connective-tissue cells, and in consequence the so-called papillæ are enlarged. Where they are free to grow—at the convex border of the cartilage, for example—they resemble little warts, or condylomata; but on the surface of the lid, where they are subjected to pressure from the cornea, they are flattened, and, being crowded against each other, form a number of irregular sulci. Such granulations are also found in chronic blennorrhœa. It is very important to recognize the difference betwen these simple granulations and trachoma bodies. In the great majority of cases, during such an acute attack, the cornea becomes inflamed—acute pannus. The trachoma keratitis will be fully described hereafter. It is sufficient to say now that the pain, photophobia, and eye distress are chiefly dependent upon the secondary keratitis.

An eye suffering from trachoma is always liable to attacks of acute inflammation. Very often the acute conjunctivitis is caused by a fresh eruption of trachoma follicles; at other times it is excited by those causes which occasion simple conjunctivitis—viz., dirt, smoke, bad air, eye-strain, etc. The acute exacerbation may last several days, even weeks, and, if not properly treated, may lead to the most disastrous ulceration of the cornea. When the cornea is not involved, the attack, although it may pass off in a few days, always leaves the eye a little more irritable than before, and more liable to a relapse. Thus the disease goes on intermittently from bad to worse, until finally there is not enough conjunctiva left to support an acute inflammation. The disease disappears, because there is no more healthy mucous membrane for it to involve.

The atrophy ends the malady, but, unfortunately, there are sequelæ, which are even more annoying than the original trouble—viz., entropion, pannus, and punctiform keratitis. It will be remembered that, in the chapter on follicular conjunctivitis, it was stated that the so-called follicles were always caused by some local irritant, which may be dust, smoke, bad air, or *trachoma bodies*. Consequently, in young eyes and many old ones a trachomatous conjunctiva may be plentifully covered with simple, non-specific follicles, so that it may be impossible for the non-expert to tell which are trachoma nodules and which are not. Such cases we call mixed—trachoma and follicular conjunctivitis. Of course, if these cases are treated for follicular conjunctivitis, they will not recover. The trachoma finally becomes apparent through the development of scar tissue, or by a most certain sign—pannus. I take it, this is the reason why some writers deny the existence of the disease follicular conjunctivitis, and unhesitatingly rank all such cases as trachoma. It is true that both diseases are very much alike in their early stages, They are both essentially chronic, but trachoma may be cured with the sulphate of copper, which will invariably make follicular ophthalmia worse. The profession has disputed, and perhaps always will dispute, the duality of the diseases.

My experience is, it is best to consider them separate diseases, for certainly a treatment based on this conclusion is the best so far discovered.

Pathology.—A trachoma body is a collection of new connective-tissue cells in the stroma of the mucous membrane, and in the substance of the cartilage immediately under the conjunctiva. It is very closely related to the infecting granulomata, but differs from them in one important respect: the cells composing the tumors do not, as in tubercle, actinomycosis, and syphilis, undergo fatty degeneration or cheesy metamorphosis but develop into connective tissue. A trachoma nodule, unless it is absorbed, which very frequently happens, necessarily destroys the tissue it involves, by implanting in it an island of scar tissue. A few such isolated scars would not interfere very much with the

function of the mucous membrane, but when the
trachoma is confluent and large areas of the conjunctiva are destroyed, serious consequences must result.
Like all cicatrizing tissue, the trachoma scar contracts;
thus it is evident that if the inner surface of the tarsal

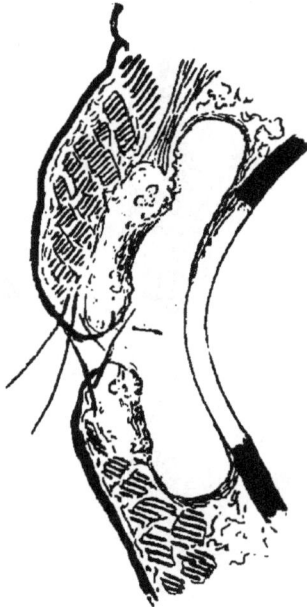

FIGURE 6.

Cross-section of the lids and cornea in an old case of trachoma, showing atrophy
of the conjunctiva, atrophy of the tarsal cartilages, and pannus.

cartilage is badly diseased, the conjunctiva covering it
will not only become atrophic, but the cartilage will be
greatly reduced in size, and, because of the contraction
on its ocular surface, it will be curved inwards. A very
familiar picture in old cases of trachoma is the deformed lid, which, when it is turned, shows a narrow
band of fleshy tissue divided longitudinally by a white
stripe. It is this apparently insignificant band of scar

tissue which plays such an important part in the changes which take place at the edge of the lid. The examiner will notice that in the normal eye the internal angle of the lid is a right angle, quite sharp, and

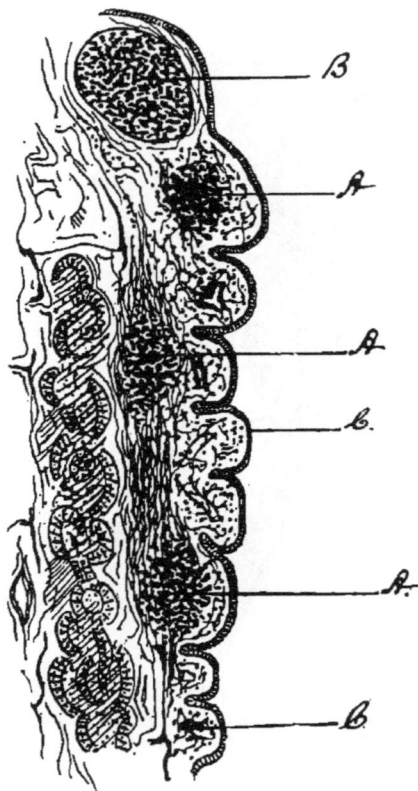

FIGURE 7.

Section of the conjunctiva of the upper lid in mixed trachoma. *A*, Trachoma bodies. *B*, Lymph follicle. *C*, Enlarged and hypertrophied so-called papillæ.

that the edge of the lid fits closely to the eyeball as it moves up and down. This angle is formed by a cushion* of mucous membrane at the extreme margin of the lid. When the conjunctiva lining the lid is destroyed,

* See Frontispiece.

the little angular cushion disappears also, so the mucous edge of the lid, instead of being square, becomes round. The mucous membrane at this place is absorbed because the scar, which runs parallel to the edge of the lid, cuts off its blood-supply. The deformity not only brings the base of the lashes nearer the eye, but it allows the curving of the upper lid to turn them downwards—entropion. The same deformity is often seen in the lower lid, when the lashes are turned upwards. The interference of the lashes of both lids in blinking when there is any degree of entropion, together with the disturbed circulation and the disease in the cartilage, excite such changes in the hair follicles that the cilia not only become diseased, but distorted, and grow out irregularly along the cutaneous edge of the lids: trichiasis, distichiasis. It is in this way that the lashes rub against the cornea.

Etiology.—The cause of trachoma is evidently a microbe, whose size, character, and history are still unknown. Some think they have found it, others deny it; at any rate, bacteriology has made it more than probable that a micro-organism is at the root of the evil. Excepting chronic blennorrhœa, trachoma is one of the most contagious diseases. Evidently the discharge contains the *materies morbi*, and it is only necessary for it to reach a conjunctival surface, prepared for its reception, to start the disease.

For a number of years I have thought that trachoma belonged to the infecting granulomata and should be classed with tubercle, actinomycosis, syphilis, etc. The trachoma body is the result of a massing of cells to destroy or isolate a foreign, irritating substance. Un-

like tubercle, the cells do not perish, but are transformed into cicatricial tissue. Consequently, if I am
correct, the disease should be most contagious in its
early and acute stages. This is found to be true, for it
is not unusual to see an entire family attacked about
the same time, yet one member of a family may be a
subject of trachomatous degeneration and none of the
others be affected. But it is a dangerous disease to
come among people in any stage. It is important to inquire, Is it necesssary for infection that the virus be
carried to the eyes by the hand, towels, or some object?
Perhaps not, for I cannot force myself to the belief that
drying the pus or secretions destroys the germs or
spores they contain. It may be true that the gonococcus
loses in part its virulency when it dries up in the secretions, for no one ever heard of gonorrhœal ophthalmia
contracted in any other way than by direct contact.
We do not take the gonorrhœa from the air, but we do
tuberculosis. We know that fresh gonorrhœal pus
is extremely infectious; yet, it is not surprising that
among the millions who suffer from gonorrhœa but a
very small per cent get ophthalmia? A very dirty,
careless fellow with acute clap may live for days in
a close cabin with a dozen or more individuals as careless and dirty as himself and not one contract ophthalmia; but let a case of trachoma or chronic blennorrhœa
come among them, and in two weeks more than half will
be diseased. The evidence is strongly in support of
the belief that the contagium can reach the eyes
through the air, and that the dried secretions are much
more dangerous than the moist. It may be said, if this
were true, none could escape, for a single individual

would infect an entire community. A few children in a family will escape scarlatina, although we know that no contagium is as persistent or certain. The probabilities are that all are not equally susceptible. It is presumptive that a healthy conjunctiva is not especially liable to contract trachoma; a diseased one is. As with children, those who have irritable, flabby throats, subject to tonsillitis, are prone to diphtheria; so in the eye: a man with chronic conjunctivitis is ready to contract either trachoma or blennorrhœa, if he has a chance; the diseased mucosa being an inviting and suitable culture-field. I do not believe trachoma runs through schools, barracks, and construction-camps because the trachoma virus is particularly virulent, but because those living in close, dirty, smoky, and foul quarters are nearly all subjects of chronic catarrhal ophthalmia.

TRACHOMATOUS KERATITIS—PANNUS.

The behavior of the cornea during the course of this disease is so varied and important that it is best at this time to consider the causes which lead to that form of keratitis we call pannus. It must be remembered that pannus is not alone peculiar to trachoma; it is seen in chronic blennorrhœa in its most aggravated form, and we will find that it is not at all uncommon in scrofulous ophthalmia. Pannus is a form of chronic superficial corneitis, characterized by a clouding of the transparent tissue and the development of blood-vessels on or near the surface of the membrane. The opacity of the cornea is caused by the deposit of inflammatory products, sometimes cells, sometimes cicatricial tissue. In describing the anatomy of the conjunctiva, I said one of the

proofs that that membrane covered the cornea was
the tendency of all chronic diseases of the conjunctiva
to encroach upon the cornea.   In trachoma it is not
at all rare to find the trachoma bodies on the eyeball;
they also invade the cornea, beginning at its edge.
When this disease attacks the cornea, it does not form
nodules, but infiltrates very similar to the little white
deposits found in the deep layers of the membrane covering the cartilage.   Such a cellular deposit may be
above Bowman's membrane or below it.   In the first
instance the neighboring epithelial layers are much
disturbed and thickened; in the latter the surrounding
cornea is inflamed.   This localized keratitis leads to
the formation of new blood-vessels, which approach the
diseased spot from the nearest conjunctival edge. Since
the disease nearly always invades the cornea from
above, the clouding and capillary development begin at
its upper border.   The trachoma infiltrate may be absorbed, frequently it generates into scar tissue, often it
breaks down into an ulcer.   If this happens before
the cornea becomes vascular, the ulcers may become
necrotic and greatly injure the eye; usually, on account
of the plentiful supply of blood from the vessels of the
pannus, they heal rapidly, but always leave indelible
scars.   This kind of pannus will form irrespective of
the condition of the lids.   When the upper lid is extensively covered by trachoma bodies and hypertrophied papillæ, so that it feels rough to the finger, it is
evident the cornea must suffer.   There results a trau-
matic, superficial keratitis and great hypertrophy of the
epithelial layer; consequently, the blood-vessels develop as in all forms of keratitis.   This may be called

friction pannus. These two forms of keratitis may arise in simple trachoma and from the two causes be combined. They are very slow in forming, but when the eye is suddenly inflamed from some extraneous cause, the corneal disease becomes aggravated. Then is the eye tender, the lids closed and swollen, and the photophobia intolerable. Every attack of this kind mars so much more the transparency of the cornea.

There is a peculiarity about the circulation in pannus which explains how it is that a cornea almost clear and anæmic can within a few hours become covered with capillaries. A blood-vessel once formed in the substance of the cornea will remain a long time. When the cause which provoked the growth of the vessel disappears, the blood ceases to circulate in it, the current stopping at the edge of the cornea. Usually one cannot see the vessel wall, so when it is empty, it is invisible. The moment the eye becomes inflamed and an irritation starts afresh in the cornea, the circulation is reëstablished. This is the only explanation I can offer for the phenomenon, for it is not possible that new capillaries can grow in so short a time. It must be noted that even in a clear cornea of one who has had a pannus a few vessels may be discerned through a magnifying-glass. In simple superficial pannus the blood-vessels come from the conjunctiva, in pannus of deep keratitis the vessels come from the episcleral plexus. It is doubtful if many cases of trachoma continue long without some pannus, but some escape severe disease of the cornea, so there may be a very badly scarred conjunctiva and yet a clear eye.

A very peculiar form of inflammation of the cornea

common in the degenerative stage of trachoma is the
punctiform keratitis, which commences, a little white
speck on the cornea, apparently in the epithelium; it
is not confined to any region of that membrane, but
may appear at any place.   It comes suddenly, and, for
a little affair, causes an immense amount of distress.
An eye which before has been comfortable suddenly
becomes injected and lachrymosed.   There is always a
great degree of photophobia.   The eye smarts; it is
painful.   When the cornea is examined, a little phlyctenule will be found.   The infiltrate always breaks down
into an ulcer, which usually penetrates Bowman's membrane.   It heals readily, if not irritated, but is apt to
be followed by others.   Then the attack may last for
weeks, and during that time the patient can scarcely
approach the light.   Sometimes these ulcers become
infected, when they grow larger and are surrounded by
a ring of inflamed cornea.   What they are and the
cause I do not know.   They are liable to attack the eye
at any time; any irritant may start them, especially
strong astringent collyria.

Whenever the cornea becomes badly inflamed in
trachoma, there is danger of iritis.

Treatment.—To treat trachoma successfully requires of the practitioner an exact understanding of the
disease, backed by experience.   When properly handled,
very much can be done for an eye, but if a mistake is
made either in the diagnosis or the treatment, irrepar-
able injury will be the result.   Trachoma is essentially
a chronic disease and requires the most careful management.   Although very much can be done for it, some
cases can only be relieved, and some cannot be con-

trolled at all. In the most hopeful cases the treatment
will last from six months to a year. A doctor may consider himself fortunate if he can *certainly* cure the disease in two years. It is the tendency to relapse which
not only annoys the attendant, but destroys the confidence of the patients. For this reason they go from one
surgeon to another. So it is unusual that one has an opportunity to handle the disease from its beginning to its
end. It is a poor man's disease, rich men have it also; to
cure it brings the doctor little more than satisfaction, to
fail injures his reputation. He secures the confidence of
a community by a brilliant piece of work, which is
undermined by the first batch of trachoma cases his
name has attracted.

The principle in the treatment is: *Reduce the disease to its simplest form, then treat it with the sulphate
of copper.* When this can be done, it can be surely
cured, but, unfortunately, it is often extremely difficult.
Some believe that the sulphate of copper is a specific
for the disease. It is possible it has no advantage over
the nitrate of silver other than it can be used longer
without straining the conjunctiva. It may be that
copper destroys the etiological organism. This can be
neither proved nor disproved. A trachoma follicle
which is slightly irritated from time to time and allowed in the intervals to remain quiescent will be absorbed. If the irritation is kept up continually, the
neoplasm will grow larger and undergo cicatricial degeneration. There is no medicine which can in any
way equal the crystal of the sulphate of copper for the
purpose of intermittent irritation. If a smooth crystal
of the salt be passed over the inverted lids, it will cause

an intense congestion of the conjunctiva; it will burn severely and the tears will flow. The irritation will last an hour or so, when the eye returns to its former condition. If the copper is rubbed on the lid, the irritation will last longer; if it is rubbed on extensively, it may cause sloughing of the mucous membrane; then, of course, the reaction will be violent and continued. So, it must be remembered that the sulphate of copper is not only an astringent, but an escharotic. The sloughs it makes are superficial; those made by the nitrate of silver may be deep. Copper is an antiseptic, but in this regard it cannot be compared to the silver salts. It is strange that the trachomatous conjunctiva, when irritated by the copper, does not usually react violently, yet it will not tolerate the irritation from particles of foreign matter. It may be said that a copper conjunctivitis is a specific inflammation which is very acute, but is soon over. As before stated, we rarely see simple trachoma in the country; it is usually mixed with other diseases, blennorrhœa and follicular conjunctivitis. These will not tolerate copper; *consequently they must be cured before the trachoma is attacked.* The treatment of chronic blennorrhœa cannot be considered here.

Given a case of simple trachoma in its early stages, wherein the mucous membrane and the retrotarsal folds are covered with soft trachoma follicles, the first thing to do is to remove as many of them as possible by surgical means, provided in doing so the conjunctiva is not extensively lacerated. The turned lid may be caught between the thumb-nails and the contents of the follicles squeezed out. We may use Knapp's roller

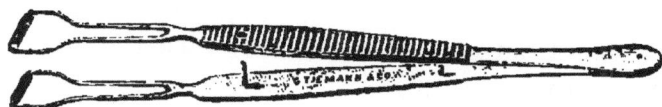

FIGURE 8.
Knapp's Forceps.

forceps and press them out. Prince's forceps are very
good and serviceable, for with them we can reach the
entire conjunctiva. With these instruments as many

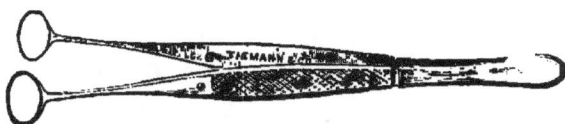

FIGURE 9.
Prince's Forceps.

of the follicles as possible must be removed, but under
no circumstances should force be used. If the disease
is in young, delicate, or nervous persons, an anæsthetic
is advisable, for the operation is painful. I prefer
beforehand to scarify very carefully the diseased surface, so that the contents of the follicles can easily escape through the cuts.

When the operation is completed, it is well to rub
over the raw surface a piece of cotton, wrapped around
a match, wet with a solution of the bichloride of
mercury 1:2000; and get as much of the antiseptic into
the tissues as possible. The lids should be covered by
a cold compress an hour or so, then the eyes let alone
for twenty-four hours, when the bichloride rubbings
should be renewed. This operation will cut short the
treatment at least four months.

The profession can never pay Doctor Hotz the debt
it owes him for the introduction of this procedure.
Disease of the cornea does not contra-indicate the opera-

—7—

tion. Indeed, it is astonishing to see how quickly the eye will get better. Some authors rather condemn it, claiming that the lacerations leave scars. That is true, but the trachoma itself will do the same and be a longer time about it. When the lids no longer bleed during the antiseptic rubbings, it is a good plan, if the inflammation does not subside, to use a mild solution of the nitrate of silver, 1 or 2 grains to the ounce, as in the treatment of simple conjunctivitis. The eyes should be protected from the light by blue glasses, and under no circumstances should the patient go about a barn or stable, or be in a place where the air is dusty or smoky. When the congestion and irritation are gone and there is no keratitis, then is the time to begin the copper treatment. Procure a good, large crystal of the sulphate of copper, file it into a convenient shape, being careful that the axis of the crayon is parallel to the axis of crystallization; then rub it on a damp towel, so that it becomes perfectly smooth; be careful that there are no sharp flaws on it. Turn the upper lid and pass the crystal over it once, then wash off the lid with a camel's-hair brush dipped in water; re-turn the lid, and let the patient bathe the eyes in cold water. The next day let the edge of the crayon go a little underneath the inverted lid. Every day make the application a little more thorough, until finally the entire diseased surface is reached. During this time watch the cornea. If it shows the slightest sign of inflammation, if it ulcerates, or a phlyctenule appears, stop the treatment immediately, for, if it is then pushed, there is danger that the cornea will become badly diseased. In such instances observe the rule, *reduce the disease again to its simplest form*, and start the copper treatment anew.   After repeated trials, the eye may be taught to stand the treatment; then it is on the rapid road to recovery.   If the eye reacts badly, either the copper cannot be used at all, or the applications are too severe. When the eye stands this treatment, the trachoma disappears, the pannus clears up, but the cornea will never again be perfectly transparent.   In some old cases of trachoma with dense pannus, even if there be no trachoma bodies on the lids, although the conjunctiva is covered with scars, the copper treatment is useful; the cornea will clear up very much, and it is possible to get fair vision.   What should be done in an attack of acute inflammatory trachoma?   My experience is, it is best to institute no active treatment, but use such gentle, soothing remedies that Nature may be assisted to hurry through the acute stage.

For the keratitis nothing can equal atropia.   Use a strong solution, 4 grains to the ounce; see that it is neutral and that when it is dropped into the eye it reaches the cornea.   To relieve the spasm of the lids, hot eye-baths are efficacious; sometimes cold are better.   If the œdema of the lids is excessive, multiple punctures with a Graefe cataract-knife are advisable.   Counter-irritation over the forehead will allay the irritability of the eye.   For this purpose use an ointment of the white precipitate of mercury in belladonna ointment, sufficiently strong to irritate the skin.   The application should be made to the skin over the eyebrows and covered with oiled silk, then a bandage.   For the lids, nothing equals a mild solution of the nitrate of silver 1 to 2 grains to the ounce.   It is well to make the application personally twice a day; but before the silver is brushed on, the surface of the inverted lid should be dried with a piece of clean blotting-paper. For some peculiar reason, in nearly all acute, painful diseases of the conjunctiva with photophobia very mild solutions of the nitrate of silver are soothing.

Trachoma can be cured without copper; the nitrate of silver will do very well. Begin this treatment by scarifying and compression, but be sure not to apply a strong solution of silver (10—15 grains to the ounce) until the cuts are well. If the mucous membrane bleeds when the lids are turned, silver is contra-indicated. *There is but one possible condition which will justify the use of silver as a cautery or an astringent on a bleeding conjunctiva—that is, ophthalmia neonatorum.*

The majority of cases of trachoma in this country are treated by silver, because they are nearly all complicated by blennorrhœa. Many physicians will ask, "What can be done for the enlarged papillæ? Is it well to cut them off?" As a rule, all operations on the mucous membrane are detrimental, excepting those already suggested. The French advise, when the superior retrotarsal folds are badly diseased, to remove them by cutting them away with curved scissors. I have done so several times, but I could not see that the operation did any good.

I see no objection to cutting off large cock's-comb papillæ, but to take a pair of scissors and trim off the hypertrophied mucosa is bad treatment. All follicular nodules and swollen papillæ left after the compression process are best let alone; they will disappear as the eye improves.

Very often during the treatment of trachoma the cornea ulcerates, which is caused either by simple trachomatous ulcers becoming infected or from the use of caustic applications. These ulcers are always angry and are apt to perforate. The infected ulcers behave like all such ulcers of the cornea; they are surrounded by a zone of inflamed and necrosed tissue, and may, if not properly treated, destroy the eye. The subjective symptoms are very severe, the photophobia so intense that the eyes cannot be properly examined without a local or general anæsthetic. The first thing to be done under such circumstances is to stop all active treatment of the conjunctiva. If using copper or a strong solution of silver, discontinue them. Either apply a 0.25 per cent solution of the nitrate of silver, or, what is better and safer, the bichloride of mercury 1:3000. Treat the cornea with atropia. If the ulcer is large, ragged, and ugly, one of two things may be done: either puncture the anterior chamber, or destroy the ulcer with the actual cautery. The simple operation of paracentesis will often give immediate relief. Thoroughly destroying the infected tissues about the ulcer with a heated platinum wire, so as to change it to a simple ulcer, is excellent treatment, but the patient must be warned of the resulting scar. The treatment of the so-called punctiform keratitis is simple. Usually we find in these cases the tarsal cartilages very much atrophied and the cornea quite clear; then the eye will not stand strong collyria. Turn the lid and either rub on it a 1:2000 solution of mercury, or make an application of a very mild solution of the nitrate of silver for its sedative effect; atropinize the eye and keep it so; protect with blue glasses, and see that all kinds of irritation are removed. If an eyelash is touching the cornea, operate on it. By this I don't mean, pluck it out, unless it is necessary. Either destroy it with electricity or transplant it. Double thread a very fine curved needle with a delicate strand of waxed silk. Enter the needle in the edge of the lid exactly where the lash comes out, curve the point upwards and outwards so that it comes out as near the normal line of the cilia as possible, pull the thread through, and engage the offending hair in the loop. That lash will not again disturb the eye.

Sometimes neither the sulphate of copper, the nitrate of silver, nor the bichloride of mercury will cure the disease; they seem to lose their effect; then it is well to try some other remedy. One of the best is the yellow oxide of mercury, especially if there is much non-inflammatory pannus. This drug is used in an ointment, 1—2 grains of the yellow oxide rubbed up in a drachm of simple cerate or vaseline. A piece of this about the size of No. 5 shot is put under the upper lid, then the lid is rubbed over the eyeball until the ointment escapes—a milky-white emulsion. This should be done once a day. If the reaction is too great, either the ointment is too strong or has been carelessly prepared; it may contain lumps of the oxide, which get entangled in the mucous membrane and burn very severely. Anything which interferes either with the movement of the lids or the drainage of the tears embarrasses the treatment. Not infrequently the trachoma attacks the mucous membrane of the lachrymal sac and canal. Then there arises a very serious complication. The epiphora keeps up an irritation of the

conjunctiva, and since one of the cardinal rules during
the treatment is to eliminate all sources of irritation,
the patency of the lachrymal passages must be established. Slit the upper canaliculus and keep the passage to the nose open by probing. Such operations
and the surgical means for the relief of entropion and
other deformities of the lids cannot be considered in
this book; they are well described in our modern text-
books.

Some fifteen years ago Dr. De Wecker, of Paris, popu-
larized the use of a Brazilian drug called jequirity, the
seed of the *Arbus precatorius*—wild liquorice. If a
cold infusion of this bean is applied to the conjunctiva, it will excite in a few hours an intense muco-
purulent inflammation, characterized by great swelling
of the lids and the formation of a croupous membrane
on the conjunctiva. The intensity of the inflammation
will depend upon the strength of the infusion and the
susceptibility of the patient. The disease lasts from
four to seven days. In some respects this is a very
reliable drug, but, if not carefully and properly used, it
may do great damage. The blennorrhœa which it
excites has the same tendency to destroy the cornea as
ordinary severe blennorrhœal ophthalmia, so in using
this drug the physician should be careful that there is
sufficient circulation in the cornea to protect it—that is,
there must be some pannus. An acute blennorrhœa
will not cure acute trachoma. But in all cases of
trachoma where the lids are scarred and there are a
few trachomatous nodules scattered over the conjunctiva the jequirity will destroy them. The cornea will
clear up remarkably, but neither jequirity nor any-

thing else will remove the scars left after corneal ulcers.
To clear the cornea and destroy the remnants of trachoma, jequirity has no advantage over copper or the yellow oxide of mercury, other than that it does so quicker.
A *slight* jequirity ophthalmia excited in an eye suffering
trachomatous degeneration, when there are repeated
attacks of punctiform keratitis, will have the happiest
effect. It should be used in the intervals between the
attacks. People who have suffered for months will be
greatly benefited; indeed, I have known numbers of
persons to be absolutely cured. Sometimes a case of
trachoma will be rebellious to ordinary treatment. If
it is then subjected to a course of jequirity, the nitrate
of silver and the sulphate of copper may be again
efficacious. But it must be remembered that under no
circumstances should jequirity be put into an eye if
there is a trace of blenorrhœa. It then acts badly, and it
is possible that the inflammation excited by the physician will get beyond his control. For this reason the
drug has fallen into disrepute. Of course, when it was
introduced and first tried in the United States it was
warmly—indeed, extravagantly—recommended. Like
all good things, it has been abused; but it has virtues
which rank it among the most valuable remedies we
have. Use a 2 per cent infusion—that is, about 10 grains
of the crushed bean to the ounce of water. Make a cold
infusion and allow it to stand 12 hours, filter through
cotton, and keep in a cool place. It should be used
when fresh. When the eye is properly prepared, turn
the upper lid and wipe it over once with a piece of
cotton wet with the medicine; wait 12 hours and see
what the effect is. If the reaction is very severe, wait

another 12 hours; if it is not, make another application, but cover more of the mucous surface. By this
time the physician should learn how much drugging
is necessary to excite quite a severe ophthalmia. The
proper degree of inflammation is, swollen lids, painful
eye, muco-purulent discharge, and a croupous membrane in the lower cul-de-sac and over the upper cartilage. When this stage is reached, about the end of 48
hours, stop the applications and leave the eye alone.
The acute stage will last about 24 hours, then quickly
subside. In one week it should be over. If this has
not cleared the cornea enough, do not try it again inside of a month. For what I may call its catalytic
effect, so valuable in trachomatous degeneration with
punctiform keratitis, a slight inflammation only is
necessary. In these cases the cornea is irritable and
there is danger of sloughing if severe ophthalmia is excited. If, from any cause, the physician becomes
alarmed, he may treat the artificial disease as suggested
in the chapter on croupous conjunctivitis.

Since the introduction of the jequirity bean, there
is no occasion to excite acute purulent ophthalmia to
clear the cornea of blinding pannus, unless it is impossible to procure the drug. For a long time it has been
recommended to subject such an eye to a course of severe
blennorrhœa by inoculating the conjunctiva with pus
from a diseased urethra or from a case of ophthalmia
neonatorum. By doing so, gonorrhœal conjunctivitis
or a disease very much like it is excited. Desperate
diseases often require heroic treatment, but the physician should think twice before doing such a thing. He
never knows, when he starts this disease, when or how

it will end; but if the eye comes through the ordeal successfully, very much is gained so far as the vision is concerned. It should not be proposed unless the pannus is thick and vascular, for there is danger that the clear cornea will slough. The pus to be used must be taken from an infant's eye in ophthalmia neonatorum; never from acute gonorrhœa. The mere suggestion is disgusting and it is dangerous, for one cannot eliminate a possible syphilitic virus nor is he sure to save the patient the constitutional sequelæ of gonorrhœa. Such an ophthalmia is dangerous to everybody brought near it; therefore, if the disease must be excited, it is advisable to use the pus from a baby's eye. The intentionally acquired disease must be treated as shown in the chapter on gonorrhœal ophthalmia.

CHAPTER XI

CHRONIC BLENNORRHŒAL CONJUNCTIVITIS.

The most common and important variety of granular lids is chronic blennorrhœa, which is nothing more than a chronic suppurative catarrh of the conjunctiva. This disease is often seen in its pure form; very frequently it is found mixed with trachoma, and, for the reasons already suggested, there will, in young people, be at the same time more or less of follicular development.

Chronic blennorrhœa usually begins as a subacute purulent conjunctivitis. At other times it is chronic from the start. In the subacute variety the eye becomes suddenly inflamed, the entire conjunctiva being involved. The lids are somewhat swollen, the eyeball very red, and there may be a slight chemosis. From the start the discharge is purulent. It will collect about the edge of the lids at night and may accumulate in the internal canthus, but never flows over the cheeks. When the lower lid is depressed, the pus can be distinctly seen in the lower cul-de-sac. It will be difficult to spring the retrotarsal folds in view because of the swelling of the lids. The mucous membrane over the superior tarsal cartilage has a velvety appearance, and it will be noticed that the cartilage is enlarged. One of the characteristic symptoms is the color of the conjunctiva. It is not bright red, as in ordinary acute catarrh, but carmine—that is, there is a blue shade in it. The eye

is painful, feels very sandy, and is suffused with tears.
This condition may last several days or weeks, when
the acute symptoms pass off, and the eye enters a stage
of chronic inflammation.   It is in this way the disease
often begins.   Sometimes an individual believes he has
caught a slight cold in the eyes and the physician may
take it for a simple catarrh.   But if he will note the
color of the inflamed area, or will turn the lid and force
the retrotarsal folds in view, there should be no doubt of
the diagnosis.   Some subacute blennorrhœas do not attack the ocular conjunctiva, but involve the membrane
covering the lids and retrotarsal folds.   But in all
cases, however slight, if the upper cul-de-sac is explored,
there will be found a purulent discharge.   Thus is the
disease ushered in; either as a subacute inflammation, or like a simple catarrh.   In the subacute stage
the inflammation is never so intense as gonorrhœal ophthalmia.   It is exactly like the disease I have called
leucorrhœal conjunctivitis.   In the mildest forms the
disease may come on so insidiously that the patient
does not know that there is anything the matter, when
suddenly from some particular cause the eyes become
acutely inflamed.   From the above it is evident that the
disease not only differs in form, but perhaps in kind.
Now, it must be distinctly remembered that chronic
blennorrhœa and trachoma are often combined in the
same eye, so there may be not only the objective and
subjective symptoms of trachoma, but also those of
blennorrhœa.   In the simple disease the trachoma
bodies are not found, but the palpebral conjunctiva
will always be covered with little papules, which give

it a velvety look, and nowhere can be seen in the membrane about the middle of the lid the little white deposits so common in trachoma. In this variety of blennorrhœa the retrotarsal folds are not much swollen, but when the lower lid is turned down, the membrane in the lower cul-de-sac will be elevated in several parallel ridges. If the patient is a child, there will be seen on the summits of these folds a few or many lymphatic follicles, which must not be mistaken for trachoma nodules; they are the result of the irritation of the blennorrhœal disease. In these cases the discharge is muco-purulent, the eyes are irritable. The patients complain that in the morning the lids are dry and seem to stick to the eyeball; that when they are rubbed and the tears flow freely, they get relief. In other cases the characteristic peculiarity is the apparent enlargement of the superior tarsal cartilages and the enormous papillary development. The mucous membrane covering the lids is greatly hypertrophied and the papillæ so large and numerous that one can understand the meaning of the term "granular ophthalmia." If in these cases the superior retrotarsal folds are forced forward, they become very prominent; are succulent, granulated, and purulent. Often there will be found a number of follicles along the convex edge of the cartilage, which may be simple follicles; the probabilities are that they are trachoma nodules.

There is another form of chronic blennorrhœa in which the inflammation is principally confined to the upper cul-de-sac. The eyes do not look inflamed, the lids may droop a little, and from time to time some muco-purulent discharge will smear the cornea and col-

lect at the edge of the lids. But the subjective symp
toms are annoying; the eyes tire easily, they are particularly sensitive to dust, smoke, and artificial light.
When they are examined, a little discharge may be
found behind the lower lid. The upper lid, when first
turned, is normal in appearance, but almost immediately colors up—it blushes. When the retrotarsal folds
are exposed, the disease is apparent. There the tissues
are decidedly inflamed and swollen, and always covered
by a quantity of purulent discharge. So far as I
know, these different forms are of one and the same
disease. With few exceptions, they begin as a subacute inflammation, then pass into chronic.

A very familiar form of sore eyes is common in this
part of the country and supposed to be contracted during harvest-time. A young man with apparently
healthy eyes starts out to make and stack hay; the
weather at the time is hot; he accidentally gets a
lot of hay-dust in his eyes, which usually happens when
he is stacking or loading. In a few hours his eyes
begin to inflame, and in a couple of days he is laid up
with an acute ophthalmia. The inflammation may be
quite severe. When the lids are examined, they are
decidedly granular and present the familiar picture of
subacute blennorrhoea. Sometimes the disease will
get well; very often it becomes chronic. If the patient
is asked the cause of his trouble, he will almost invariably say that he got hay-dust in his eyes. Many times
there is no doubt that he is correct, but often the
patient before the accident had a chronic blennorrhoea,
and the irritation of the sharp particles of hay-fiber
excited an acute exacerbation.

Because of the relation of the surface of the cornea
to the conjunctiva, and because in all blennorrhoeal
diseases the epithelial surface suffers the most, this disease is particularly prone to attack the cornea. We see
exfoliation of the epithelium, superficial or deep ulcers,
keratitis, and acute inflammatory pannus. But these
lesions are not so common in the early stages as later,
when the conjunctiva has suffered permanent damage.
The cornea will not inflame in the initial attack unless
the disease is neglected or badly handled. It is during
the acute exacerbations which come from time to time

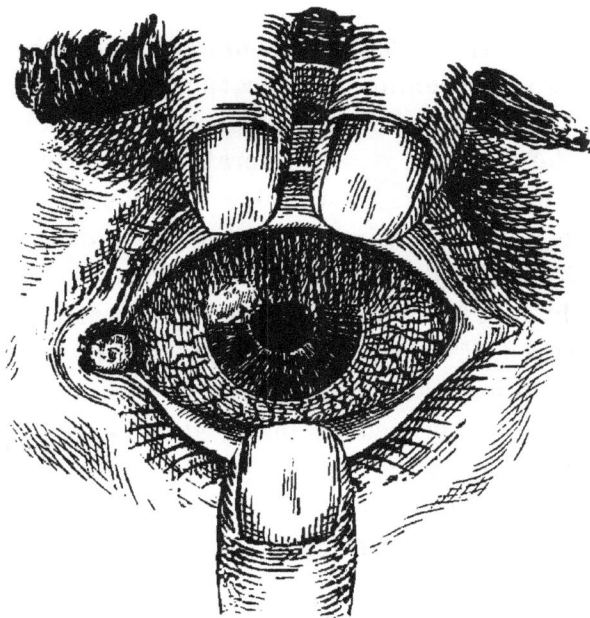

FIGURE 10.

A drawing to show the appearance of the eyeball in the acute keratitis of
chronic blennorrhœa—acute pannus--ulcer of the cornea.

in the course of the disease when arises the annoying and dangerous keratitis. Every doctor is famil-

iar with the appearance of the cornea in the bad attacks
of acute inflammation occurring during harvest-time.
Unlike the pannus in trachoma, the blood-vessels do
not come particularly from the upper part of the eye,
but from the entire circumference of the cornea.   In
this disease, as in trachoma, very much of the clouding
in the cornea is caused by scars left from ulcers, but it
must be remembered that during the acute attack the
clouding and vascularization of the cornea is not pannus, but keratitis, which will, to a certain extent, mar
its transparency.   It is not as dangerous as it looks,
but, unfortunately, if the keratitis is very severe, there
is danger of iritis.   The great danger arises from the
inflammatory softening of the cornea, when it gives to
the intraocular tension and bulges out—keratoglobus.
One of the dangers of acute keratitis in chronic blennorrhœa is extensive ulceration.   One would believe
that the unnatural circulation in the cornea would
protect it, but it does not.   The cornea may be almost destroyed by ulcers.   My experience is, even after the disease is cured, it may be a long time before the ulcers
heal.   In a few cases of chronic blennorrhœa the skin at
the edge of the lids becomes inflamed and excoriated because of the irritating discharge; then it will be seen
that the follicles at the roots of the cilia are also diseased.   There is a suppurative blepharociliaris.   As the
disease progresses the lashes fall out and the cutaneous
edge of the lid becomes pitted with ulcers—chronic
suppurating eczema.   If the conjunctiva over the
lower lid and in the inferior cul-de-sac is swollen
enough to push the edge of the lid away from the eye
and displace the lower punctum, the tears will not run

into the nose, but will bathe the already diseased lid, which, of course, makes the blepharitis worse. In time the eczematous area contracts and turns the lid out. The ectropion thus started completes a vicious circle. So it happens that in some old cases of blennorrhœa the lids are rolled out and covered by a red, inflamed, granulating mucosa.

In nearly all cases of chronic blennorrhœa the external canthus is more or less deformed. If the physician will examine the normal eye, he will see that at the external canthus the junction of the lids is an acute angle, sharp and well defined, which is true both of the skin edge and the mucous edge. When a discharge continually moistens the skin at the canthus, a small excoriation or ulcer forms, which ultimately becomes a true fissure. It is quite painful and prevents the lids being opened fully, and in young persons causes blepharo-spasm. After the fissure has lasted some time, it heals by second intention, when, of course, the skin is drawn over the canthus—a vertical band pulling both on the skin of the upper and lower lids. In the great majority of cases this little deformity is harmless, but since it has a tendency to prevent the lids being properly opened, and sometimes assists in rolling under the lids in entropion, it may become a matter of importance.

Although the pathology of chronic blennorrhœa is simple (Chapter III.), there are some clinical peculiarities which are noteworthy. In some cases of chronic blennorrhœa of the conjunctiva the mucous membrane rapidly atrophies, and there is an early formation of cicatricial tissue. In other cases, exactly of the same kind, the membrane may be inflamed a long time before

—8—

it becomes permanently damaged. Then the inner surfaces of the lids are covered by scar tissue; never so great, however, as in trachoma. It is doubtful if pure chronic blennorrhœa leads to sufficient cicatricial changes to deform the lids by contraction. All it will do in the worst cases is to destroy the mucous function of the conjunctiva.

Before considering the cause of this disease, it is well to examine the character of blennorrhœas in general, since bacteriology has completely negatived all that has been written concerning them up to a few years ago. A mucous membrane may suppurate from one of two causes: 1. It may be invaded by micro-organisms, which live and grow on and in it. These cause an exudation of pus. Such an organism is the gonococcus, which may be considered the king coccus of all true blennorrhœas. Let it be remembered that the mucous membrane of the eye, vagina, urethra, and rectum are suitable nourishing media for this organism. When it attacks them, it will multiply indefinitely unless the culture is destroyed by a drug, ptomaïn, antitoxin, or phagocytes. It is not stretching the imagination to reason that the gonococcus is the result of a long period of evolution; that its ancestor was a micro-organism, which found the genital mucosa a fitting medium for its propagation; and is it at all improbable if we say that the virulent character of that organism is lessened when it is in the process of degeneration? Thus it is, I believe, that the micro-organisms which cause all forms of true blennorrhœal ophthalmia have either a gonorrhœal ancestry or are nearly related to it in the process of evolution. Such micro-organisms cause

true blennorrhœa. 2. All other forms of blennorrhœa
I shall call false. They are the results of a secondary
infection by the ordinary surgical pus microbes, the
streptococci, staphylococci, etc. These micro-organisms
do not flourish on or under mucous epithelium; their
presence will inflame a mucous membrane, but such an
inflammation is catarrhal; the leucocytes are killed
after they reach the surface, not before, as in true
blennorrhœa.

A very good example of this disease is found in
the conjunctivitis accompanying chronic suppurative
dacryocystitis. In these instances the fluid in the
lachrymal sac is a culture of the pyogenic cocci which
reach it from the eye. This fluid contains myriads of
micro-organisms, and is, of course, a concentrated solution of toxines. The discharge is especially irritating
to the conjunctiva and causes the conjunctivitis. If it
reaches the connective-tissue stroma, it immediately
causes a diffuse cellulitis. Abscess in the soft parts
about the lacrymal sac and abscess of the cornea are
often excited in this manner. Now, however severely
the conjunctiva may be inflamed, as soon as the diseased sac is cleaned and drained the ophthalmia disappears. Exactly in this way is an otorrhœa started
and continued. The discharge from the ear is a false
blennorrhœa and the result of secondary infection, for,
however severe the otorrhœa may be, it will stop as soon
as the middle ear is drained and cleaned. Ordinary
pus, therefore, will not excite blennorrhœal conjunctivitis. There is one exception: pus from the urethra
or vagina will.

In giving the causes of ophthalmia neonatorum I

called attention to the fact that although gonorrhœa
was often responsible, still there were times when there
could not possibly be found any connection between the
two diseases.   The same was said regarding leucorrhœal ophthalmia.   If the discharges from simple
leucorrhœa can cause acute and subacute blennorrhœal
conjunctivitis, they may also cause chronic; so it is very
probable that from this source we get the contagium
which is responsible for one variety of granular lids.
My experience leads me to suspect that there is something in hay-dust which will excite acute granular
conjunctivitis.   It may be that it is a microbe, or it is
the sharp particles of dried fiber, which excite the
irritation.   That such dust will inflame an eye is certainly true, for I have seen many cases of conjunctivitis
directly caused by it—at least, I think so.   It must not
be presumed that every case of granular lids with such
a history is caused by that irritant.   Many farmers
have a chronic blennorrhœal conjunctivitis and do not
know it.   If such eyes are severely irritated in the
harvest-field, the acute inflammation is but an exacerbation of the chronic disease.

The discharge from a chronic blennorrhœal eye is
remarkably contagious.   There are but few people
immuned.   Whether the contagium reaches the eye
dried or moist, the result is the same, although it is possible that fresh pus is more virulent than stale.   But
the proofs are so conclusive that it may be safely
affirmed that most cases are contracted through the
air, for it is impossible to believe that half the men in
a railroad construction-camp car will be infected by a
single individual and from one another by immediate

contact. Usually it is the dried discharge disseminated
through the atmosphere which is responsible for the
outbreaks of chronic blennorrhœa we so often see in
barracks, camps, prisons, and schools.

Persons suffering from chronic blennorrhœal conjunctivitis have decidedly weak eyes. They complain
that using the eyes for any purpose hurts them. They
smart, are sandy and very uncomfortable. On waking
in the morning the eyes feel particularly dry, which is
not relieved until the lids are rubbed and the tears
flow. The lids are usually glued together during sleep,
or there will form a collection of dried discharge at the
base of the lashes. From time to time during the day
the discharge smears the cornea, the vision is blurred,
which only lasts a moment, for the patient instinctively
rubs the eye and clears the cornea. Their eyes are easily irritated; the act of the accommodation in reading
congests the eyeball, and such slight irritations, which
would not disturb a healthy eye, quickly inflame them.
If the cornea is not diseased, they do not suffer much
pain; but if there is the slightest keratitis, the photophobia may be very distressing. Usually the subjective symptoms are not more severe than in ordinary
subacute catarrh.

The Prognosis of ordinary simple chronic blennorrhœa is reasonably good—that is, if the patient
gets the right treatment; otherwise it is bad, for very
few cases get well unassisted. Some eyes cannot be
cured; fair-skinned, red-headed people make very bad
subjects. The prognosis again depends very much
upon the patient's business, surroundings, and the
ability to remain under treatment. Farmers suffer

when they have blennorrhœal ophthalmia because they are continually exposed to the bright sun, changeable air, and barn-dust. I believe it impossible to cure any one who continues to work about a stable. It takes time, often a long time, to cure this disease; so many who practice in large cities do not often succeed, because so few patients from the country have the means to remain until they are well. Our most hopeful patients are of the wealthy class, who have the time and conveniences to assist the oculist. The behavior of the cornea influences the prognosis very much. Extensive keratitis is a grave complication; ulcers very readily become infected, and may eat into the anterior chamber. Simple pannus, even if the cornea be covered with blood-vessels, is not as bad as it looks. It will clear up very rapidly as the disease in the conjunctiva improves, but it must not be forgotten that if the patient is blind, the cornea will never again be perfectly transparent; the sight may improve very much, but it is rare that the vision will be good enough for reading.

Iritis secondary to perforation of the cornea, or severe keratitis, nearly always occludes the pupil, but if the physician recognizes this complication in time and starts immediately to dilate the pupil with a strong mydriatic, the eye may be saved. As before stated, the prognosis depends a great deal upon the proficiency of the oculist and the docility of the patient. These cases, if treated badly, will invariably get worse.

Treatment.—If it will be remembered that the majority of people suffering from disease of the eye in this part of our country have chronic blennorrhœal conjunctivitis, it is evident that the chapter on the treatment of this disease is the most important in the book. The proper management of these cases is extremely difficult, for the doctor will find that no particular line of treatment will cure all. A drug that will benefit one eye may destroy another, and until one has had much experience he canot tell, until he tries, what will be good and what will be bad. Again, the patient himself is often responsible for the failure in his case, for he cannot understand that a chronic disease is hard to control; so he usually goes from one oculist to another and gives none an opportunity to effect a cure.

This disease is caused by a microbe, which lives and multiplies in the mucous membrane. To cure it, one must remove the cause, either by destroying it or assisting Nature to do so. The treatment, therefore, is essentially anti-bacterial. Now, it is not difficult to destroy a culture of micro-organisms if it can be reached, but, unfortunately, the antiseptic which kills the germs often destroys the tissue they inhabit. When a small area is involved, as in infected ulcer of the cornea, the actual cautery is very effective, for the doctor can afford to destroy a part of the cornea to save the whole. But there is no time in chronic blennorrhœa when the disease is limtied to a small area of the conjunctiva; it is usually diffused over the entire membrane. It is evident, therefore, that an antiseptic, even if very powerful, must be brought in contact with the whole diseased surface. Powerful antiseptics are not applicable, for two reasons: they destroy the conjunctiva, and they disease the cornea. If it were not so, one could fill the conjunctival sac with an antiseptic

powder or ointment and cure the case in a very few
days. If the bacterial colony were on the surface of
the membrane, continued mild antiseptic washes would
be effective; but the microbes are under the epithelium.
A wash that could reach and destroy them would be
stronger than the eye would bear. If we could cure a
blennorrhœa at the risk of injuring to a certain extent
the conjunctiva, there are times when we would not hesitate to do so, but we cannot then avoid endangering
the integrity of the cornea. In cases of chronic blennorrhœa when the cornea is covered by a vascular
pannus, which to a certain extent protects it, it is found
that the applications of a strong antiseptic act quickly,
certainly, and harmlessly. It is fortunate that a mild
antiseptic which will not destroy a multitude of microbes will retard their growth. If a culture in the substance of the mucous membrane can be thus held in
check, the phagocytes will soon remove them and Nature effect a cure. That can be done without irritating
the cornea. It is on this principle that the modern
treatment is based. Our endeavors should be to destroy and remove all the germs possible, and at the
same time paralyze those deep in the tissue so that they
cannot resist the attack of the white corpuscles.

Let me say here, there is no specific for chronic
blennorrhœa. What peculiar power the sulphate of
copper has beyond its irritating effect on trachoma
I do not know; for that disease it is a specific, but
for chronic blennorrhœa it is useless—indeed, often
harmful.

The choice of antiseptic methods to employ in the
disease depends upon the peculiarities and character

of the case. As I have endeavored to show, chronic blennorrhœal conjunctivitis behaves differently in different people. In some cases there is found more of the trouble at the superior cul-de-sac, in others the tarsal part of the mucosa is chiefly involved, then again the entire conjunctiva may be affected. The treatment, therefore, will depend very much upon the character of the case.

The two antiseptics chiefly employed are the nitrate of silver and the bichloride of mercury. The silver salt has the advantage that it is not only a powerful antiseptic, but it is also an astringent. It is used in strengths ranging from 1 to 30 grains to the ounce of water. A mild solution dropped into the eye three times a day will keep the conjunctival sac aseptic, but it has no penetrating power. A strong solution cannot be applied to the entire conjunctiva as a collyrium, it must be penciled on the inner surface of the lids, and then neutralized.

When a strong solution of the nitrate of silver is applied to a blennorrhœal mucous surface, it immediately penetrates the membrane. The silver salt first coagulates the albumen on the surface and between the epithelial cells; it also destroys the protoplasm of the cells—it kills them. Thus is formed a coagulum of the albuminate of silver which has imprisoned in it a quantity of dead epithelium and myriads of micro-organisms that are killed by the antiseptic. In forming the coagulum some of the nitrate of silver is used up, and consequently the strength of the solution is reduced; the salt still penetrates, the coagulation

and the destruction of the soft tissues go on, but
finally stop when the solution is no longer strong
enough to precipitate the intercellular fluids.   But
there is a little silver left, which acts as a mild but
sure antiseptic.   In this way it is possible to reach the
deep parts of the membrana propria, and destroy or
paralyze *in situ* the septic organisms.   In a few hours
the superficial coagulum melts away or is thrown off
because of the reaction of the underlying tissues and
the exudation of serum.   In the meantime the phagocytes have destroyed or carried away the dead or torpid
germs; the surface covers over again with new epithelium, when it can be said that part of the membrane is
less septic than before!   A solution of from 10 to 20
grains to the ounce will act in this manner.   Stronger
solutions penetrate too deeply and destroy too much of
the mucous connective tissue; they make a false membrane very much like diphtheria, which must slough off
and is apt to leave an ulcer.   There are two reasons why
the nitrate of silver cannot always be used in this way:
1. It is impossible to make such an application to the
entire conjunctiva.   That part which has not been
cauterized will soon reinfect that which has, for a second application cannot be made until the effects of the
first are gone.   2. Such treatments are very irritating,
and the inflammation excited in the conjunctiva will
react on the cornea.   Those who have used strong solutions of silver have noticed how often the cornea ulcerates.   But, for all that, the nitrate of silver is extremely valuable.

The antiseptic properties of the bichloride of mercury make it a very useful drug in blennorrhœa, since

more can be done with it than any other single remedy. For that particular form of the disease for which silver is useful it is not so good, but there are many cases it will cure which cannot be treated by silver. It has one advantage over the nitrate of silver—it can be used longer, and it does not stain the conjunctiva. The yellow oxide of mercury is another very valuable antiseptic. It is particularly useful because it can be used in an ointment and thus retained longer in the conjunctival sac than solutions. I have no faith in sulphate of copper solutions or simple astringents. Tannic acid, boro-glycerin mixtures, compounds of the zinc and copper salts containing some vegetable extract are, in my opinion, useless. If they do good at all, they do so by keeping the eye clean. Although they are useless, yet they are dangerous, for they all irritate and inflame the cornea. The reader should not forget that for the successful treatment of this disease the conjunctival sac must be kept clean and the eye protected from all kinds of irritation. Even the irritation from the medicinal applications is bad. That must happen, so he should do all in his power to relieve, by soothing means, that which he has excited by remedies; nor should the physician forget that while he is an oculist he is a doctor. Internal drugging will sometimes help very much; a weak anæmic man wants tonics, cod-liver oil, fresh air. Such patients should be out of doors as much as possible; nothing can be more detrimental than close, foul air. Clean clothes and a clean skin help to clean an eye. Cheerful surroundings and hope stimulate the tissue cells to do their part quickly and

well.   If the patients are sick, they must be relieved.
It would be impossible to cure a chronic blennorrhoeal
conjunctivitis in an individual suffering from diabetes
with excessive glycosuria without internal medication.
No surgeon would attempt to operate on such an one
until, by diet and medicines, he had reduced the loss of
the sugar and elevated the body tone.   It is well, in
adults, to look to the kidneys.   The confinement and
forced indolence which many of these patients suffer before they reach the oculist often excite lithæmia.   The
urine is then highly colored, scanty, and charged with
the products of imperfect assimilation, urates and uric
acid.   Then will a little dilute nitro-muriatic acid, and
less nitrogenous food, together with exercise, do wonders.   True, the disease is purely local; but, as I said
before, one can only assist the body to throw it off, to
do which he must act both on the surface and through
the blood.

When the disease is limited to the mucous membrane forming the superior retrotarsal folds, and there
is no thickening of the tarsal conjunctiva, the best
treatment is the local application of the nitrate of silver, the stronger the solution the better.   It may
be from 20 to 30 grains to the ounce.   The object is
to destroy the redundant tissues and kill by such a
powerful antiseptic the septic germs which are imprisoned in the depressions and pockets of the inflamed
membrane.   To make the application requires the help
of an assistant.   The upper lid is turned and held by
the thumb of the left hand, the patient is directed to
look down; then, through the lower lid, the eyeball is
pushed inward and upwards by the thumb of the right

hand. If there is any swelling of the tissues above the upper lid, they will immediately spring into view. While the surgeon holds the lids, an assistant rapidly dries the prolapsed folds of membrane with a piece of clean blotting-paper. Then, with a camel's-hair brush, he (the assistant) should carefully apply the silver to the diseased surface. After waiting until the parts turn white and the solution penetrates, he must neutralize the caustic with salt water. If the application is properly made, there is no danger of any of the solution touching the eyeball. The treatment will cause some smarting, but not enough to distress the patient.

Such an application should be made every day or every other day until the diseased mucosa is cured. It is surprising to see how quickly the eye will improve; patients who have suffered for months may be well in a few days. It is not necessary to do anything more for the eye, but the boracic wash, used two or three times a day, will be particularly soothing. In these cases the eye is irritated by the toxines and discharges which continually come from above. The silver salt destroys the nests of septic germs in the superior cul-de-sac. Sometimes it happens that the physician cannot expose the folds, or he has no assistant; then the patient can push his eye upwards and inwards with his forefinger. The success of the treatment will depend upon the ability of the surgeon to reach the entire suppurating surface. In young people, when the folds are exposed, they may be found covered by soft lymphatic follicles. Then it is best to remove them by compression or with Knapp's or Prince's forceps.

In diffused chronic blennorrhœal conjunctivitis when the entire conjunctiva takes part in the suppurating process, in those cases where the upper lids and cartilages are enlarged and the mucous membrane covering them is thick, succulent, and papillary, the nitrate of silver is sometimes efficacious, but it should be used in a mild solution, 5 to 10 grains to the ounce, and should be applied to the conjunctiva lining the lids and the superior and inferior folds. My experience is, for the majority of such cases, the silver is useless. The best treatment is local bleeding (scarification) and the application of the bichloride of mercury. Scarifying the conjunctiva is almost a lost art. Let it be revived, for there is nothing more beneficial than local bleeding in these cases.

The object in bleeding is to keep the inflamed tissues bathed in fresh arterial blood. When a mucous membrane becomes invaded by millions of septic organisms, it begins the battle by bringing to the parts all the blood it can hold. At first the circulation is free, but as inflammatory changes take place, it becomes embarrassed because of the pressure on the venous radicles which leads to passive congestion.

If the white blood-corpuscles act as phagocytes, it is evident that when they are exhausted or hold within themselves captured organisms, they must leave the field of action and give way to fresh corpuscles or they will succumb. At this time the lymph channels and veins are choked with stagnant fluids, hindering their absorption. If the blood serum is an active agent in the contest, the same reasoning holds good, for it is evident, the greater the amount of fresh blood in the tissues the

quicker the contest will be decided.   To a culture of
micro-organisms fresh blood serum is destructive; to
the same host stale serum is nutritious.   The connective-tissue cells probably take no active part in the contest; they simply react to the irritation, multiply, and
as neutrals embarrass the field of action, although in
some forms of inflammation they serve to imprison
the offending irritants, as in some of the infecting
granulomata—trachoma, for instance.   If the used-up
blood cannot be forced back into the circulation, it
can be removed, and a fresh supply permitted to take
its place; scarification will do this.

It is probable a mild solution of corrosive sublimate has an inhibitory influence on the growth of micro-
organisms; it is certain that in living tissues only strong
solutions will kill them.   To use the bichloride of
mercury to destroy them on the surface of the conjunctiva is impracticable, for it would not only kill
the cocci, but necrose the tissues; consequently it is not
safe to use solutions stronger than 1 to 2000.   Even
then, it is necessary to be guarded, for such solutions
may be very irritating.   This medicine, in appropriate
strength, must be brought in contact with the *entire diseased* surface, and it should be forced in between the
epithelial cells.   When the surface of the diseased
membrane is attacked by this agent and the deep parts
continually bathed in fresh arterial blood, the septic
germs will have a poor chance to thrive.   They will
ultimately disappear.

To scarify the conjunctiva seems a simple matter,
but to do it properly is a delicate surgical operation.   It
is not necessary to cut deep into the mucous mem-

brane; only the most superficial incisions should be
practiced, and they should be made with the point of a
sharp knife. The cuts should not be more than one-
eighth of an inch long, and not deeper than necessary
to reach the blood.   They should be mere scratches,
yet incisions.   It is not essential nor practical to scarify
the lower lids, nor should the ocular conjunctiva be
wounded.   Attack alone the upper lid, and let the field
of operation extend as far towards the upper cul-de-sac
as possible.   Use a Graefe cataract-knife with a sharp,

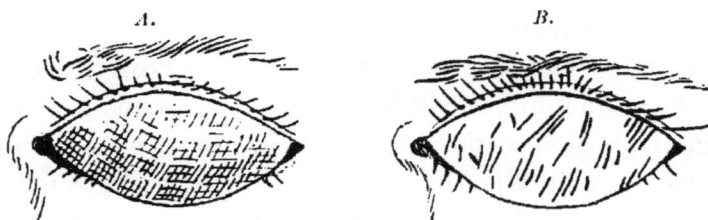

FIGURE 11.

A, The appearance of the inverted upper lid when correctly scarified. *B*, The
same carelessly, badly done.

narrow point, and, holding the instrument like a pen,
start the scarification at the lower edge of the inverted
lid, so that as the blood flows it does not hide the field
of operation.   In this way the entire surface of the lid
should be gone over; but as the free edge is approached
the cuts should be smaller and scattered, for at that
part of the lid the conjunctiva, even when inflamed, is
very thin.   A plentiful flow of blood should be en-
couraged. Unfortunately, the operation is painful, but
may be made bearable by cocaine.

When the bleeding stops, apply to the conjunctiva of both lids a solution of the bichloride, in salt
water, 1 to 2000.   It should be gently rubbed on the

membrane by a cotton applicator; a piece of absorbent cotton wrapped around the end of a match or toothpick will do very well. These applications should be made once a day, and roughly enough to make the wounded membrane bleed afresh. Twenty-four hours after the operation a false membrane will be formed on the upper lid, which should be rubbed off by the applicator moistened with the antiseptic. In a few days the membrane will not bleed when rubbed. Then the lids will be much thinner. The discharge will gradually cease. If there is any swelling, scarify again. It is rarely necessary to do so more than three times. Between the daily treatments it is well to wash out the eye with a solution of the bichloride 1 to 5000 or the boracic acid wash. It is astonishing to see how rapidly the eye will recover; not infrequently the disease will be cured in two or three weeks. When the scarifications have been properly done, the lids will heal without scars. It is not necessary to interfere with the cornea; as the eye improves that membrane will improve also. If it is very opaque from keratitis, it will not clear up completely, although, after the disease is cured, a course of jequirity ophthalmia may materially aid vision.

Of course, it is to be understood that atropia is indicated in all cases where there are any signs of keratitis. Sometimes during the treatment, the bichloride seems to lose its effect; then I would advise several applications of a 1 per cent solution of the nitrate of silver, which must be carefully washed off; but under no circumstances should the silver be used if the conjunctiva shows any tendency to bleed.

9-

The third form of chronic blennorrhœa, characterized by a mild inflammation of the entire conjunctiva,
where there is not much hypertrophy of the membrane,
the cartilages not markedly swollen and the lids
smooth; those cases in which, when the lower lid is
depressed, the conjunctiva from the inferior cul-de-sac
comes forward in parallel folds between which is seen
some pus, are very difficult to cure. My experience is,
the nitrate of silver has no effect whatever. The best
treatment is the bichloride rubbings; scarifying is unnecessary, but the application should be quite roughly
made, and for that purpose nothing is better than prepared cotton-wool* wrapped around the end of a match.
The treatment may last for weeks before the eye shows
improvement.

However greatly one may be experienced in the
management of granular lids, there are times when he
will be compelled to use empirical means, for it cannot be denied that some cases of blennorrhœa cannot be
cured by the treatment above suggested. Then it is
advisable to try the astringents. For a number of
years there was used quite a favorite prescription.
It was a solution of the sulphate of zinc, sulphate of
copper, and alum in glycerin and water. It was a
dreadful mixture to put in the eye, but it had the
reputation of curing many cases, though there were
thousands it did not cure. In the chapter on mixed trachoma it will be seen that there are conditions where
such a mixture is advisable. It may cure simple chronic

---

*Cotton-wool is finely prepared wool used by surgeons in porous dressings.
It has more body to it than cotton, and cannot be compressed into a hard
wad. When it is wrapped around the end of a match, it makes a most excellent applicator, if slight roughness is desired.

blennorrhœa. When all other rational treatment fails, the mixture of the compound astringents may be tried; but I would advise the doctor to watch carefully the cornea and stop it as soon as any keratitis arises, which will happen in the majority of cases. Sometimes an ointment of tannic acid acts well and rapidly. There is no danger of injuring the eye with this medicine, so the ointment may be made any strength. I have found that the yellow oxide of mercury ointment will do good sometimes, not often. Tannic acid mixed with the sugar of milk dusted into the eye with a camel's-hair brush has been used with effect. I have, on suggestion, rubbed the surface of the inverted lids with powdered boracic acid, but I could not see that it did any good.

Wells, our Belgian authority, advised rubbing the lid with the acetate of lead, and claimed that it did wonders. The treatment is almost forgotten; it is presumptive that it, too, has gone the way of others once extravagantly extolled, tried, then abandoned; so with hundreds of others, among which were iodoform, antipyrin, etc.

MIXED TRACHOMA.

One of the reasons why ordinary granulated lids is so difficult to cure is, it is usually a mixture of trachoma and blennorrhœa. From what has been said above, it should not be difficult for the reader to understand the pathology of this disease and picture to himself the appearance of the lids and conjunctiva. It is one of two things, either blennorrhœa has attacked a trachomatous eye or trachoma a blennorrhœal eye. Usually the latter, for if the infections were mixed, the

suppurative inflammation would be the first established. Be that as it may, the two are associated, and
if the practitioner does not recognize it, his treatment
will be ineffectual. In these cases the blennorrhœa
must be cured first, then the trachoma. Again, the
fundamental principle is emphasized: *Reduce the
trachoma to its simplest form, then treat with the sulphate
of copper.* The first step is, remove all the soft trachoma nodules and enlarged follicules by surgical
means, keep the eye clean until the inflammatory reaction is gone, using a wash of the bichloride of mercury.
1:4000. Then examine and see if the blennorrhœa is
confined to the upper cul-de-sac; if so, attack it with a
strong solution of the nitrate of silver. If the disease
involves extensively the lids, scarification is in order,
followed by the bichloride treatment. When by these
means the blennorrhœa is stopped, try an application
of the crystal of copper. If the eye stands it and the
blennorrhœa does not return, continue the copper
treatment.

It will require from six months' to three years' careful attention to cure such cases. Even then, some will
resist all our endeavors, for there are patients who
cannot be cured.

GRANULATED LIDS.

Recapitulation.—The term "granulated lids" can
mean either of the three diseases: trachoma, chronic
blennorrhœa, or follicular conjunctivitis. Trachoma,
uncontaminated by blennorrhœa or follicular catarrh,
is called simple trachoma. It is rarely seen in this
western country. The best remedies for it are the

sulphate of copper, the nitrate of silver, or the bichloride of mercury. Trachoma is nearly always found in this country mixed with blennorrhœal conjunctivitis or follicular catarrh, or both. Then it is necessary to cure the conjunctivitis or catarrh and reduce the disease to its simplest form. When that is done, the best final treatment is the sulphate of copper.

Chronic Blennorrhoea is a purulent conjunctivitis. The inflammation may involve the entire conjunctiva, or it can be limited to the fold of the mucous membrane in the upper cul-de-sac. Of diffused purulent conjunctivitis, there are two varieties. In one the conjunctiva lining the lids and making the retrotarsal folds is inflamed, but not particularly thickened; it is carmine-colored, and slightly velvety. In the other, the entire mucous membrane is thick, succulent, and the papillæ on the cartilages very numerous and large. In the first the ocular conjunctiva is not apt to be inflamed and the cornea is usually clear. In the second the eyeball is always red and the cornea liable to become diseased. When the inflammation is limited to the superior retrotarsal folds, the eyes are not injected and the conjunctiva lining the lids looks healthy, but as soon as the upper lids are turned, they become congested—that is, they blush. If the superior cul-de-sacs are explored, it will be found that the swollen and infiltrated mucosa is covered by a purulent discharge. Such eyes are irritable and easily inflamed; there is apt to be slight ptosis. Blennorrhœa of all kinds must be treated antiseptically. The best remedies are the nitrate of silver and the bichloride of mercury. *The sulphate of copper will make the disease worse, and will almost surely inflame the cornea.*   Consequently the student will appreciate the advisability of attacking the blennorrhœa first in cases of mixed trachoma.

Follicular Conjunctivitis is a catarrhal disease caused by some local irritant.   It may be dust, smoke, bad air, strain of the accommodative apparatus, blennorrhœa, or trachoma.   The treatment is to remove the cause if possible, and to empty the follicles by compression. For simple follicular conjunctivitis, when there are but few follicles and an operation is unnecessary or impossible, I think the best local remedy is a collyrium of the acetate of lead—that is, provided the cornea is healthy.

CHAPTER XII.

DIPHTHERITIC CONJUNCTIVITIS.

One of the most dreadful diseases which can attack the eye is diphtheria. This disease of the conjunctiva is, fortunately, very rare in this country, for, in my experience in Missouri, I have only seen a few cases. There are many practitioners who have never seen any, and there are thousands of medical men who would be puzzled to make the diagnosis if they did see it. This is not to be wondered at, for, until Von Graefe described the disease in the fifties, it was without a name.

The inflammation starts like an acute conjunctivitis —congestion of the eye, the sandy feeling, and pain. Within a few hours the lids, the upper especially, grow oedematous; they swell enormously, get hot, and very hard. The pain is so great that it is impossible to move them without causing much suffering. Even under an anaesthetic the doctor will have difficulty in turning them. Of course, the upper lid hangs over the lower as in gonorrhoeal ophthalmia. From the eye flows a little serous discharge, which may contain flakes of yellowish-white material as in croupous ophthalmia.

If the examiner can gently raise the lid a little by grasping the lashes, he may get a view of a part of the conjunctiva, and may see a little of the under surface of the upper lid, where he is apt to find a false membrane. In some cases the lids are so swollen and indurated that, without an anæsthetic, it is impossible to see the cornea; at other times, when the amount of diphtheritic deposit is limited, it is possible to see the eye. When the eye can be examined and the false membrane seen, there should be no difficulty in making the diagnosis, for there is a dirty-white membrane intimately adherent to a thick, dense, inflamed mucosa. The conjunctiva around the diphtheritic spot is so anæmic from plastic infiltrations that it has a waxy look, but that part of the membrane distant from it is red and engorged, and may bleed a little. If the false membrane is on the ocular conjunctiva, there will be considerable chemosis, as in acute purulent ophthalmia, and it will be noticed that near or adjoining the false membrane the cornea is hazy. The discharge will contain very little, if any, pus. Such is the usual condition of the eye on the second or third day. The constitutional symptoms depend upon the condition of the patient and the severity of the inflammation. If the disease attacks a patient suffering from fauceal diphtheria, the symptoms will be exaggerated; if it attacks the eye of one free of diphtheria, the symptoms may be marked, but not necessarily severe. In all cases there will be the systemic disturbances of diphtheria—viz., fever, rapid pulse, depression, and, because of the pain and the anxiety necessarily associated with such a fearful ophthalmic disease, restlessness.

When the disease has reached its acme, which lasts from two to three days, the objective symptoms change. The lids become softer, the local fever leaves them, and the discharge changes to a flow of pus. At this time it simulates exactly acute purulent ophthalmia.

As soon as the lids soften and can be turned, the damage that has been done can be appreciated. Every bit of the conjunctiva involved in the false membrane will be destroyed. Here and there will be seen the remnants of the deposit which has not entirely sloughed off. In other places the mucous membrane presents ragged, flat ulcers, which are bathed in pus and bleed if disturbed. The cornea may be totally destroyed. Usually it will be deeply ulcerated, somewhere between its center and its periphery. As a rule, the ulcer reaches the edge of the conjunctiva. This, the decline of the disease, lasts from one to two weeks. The suppuration gradually ceases; the ulcers heal by granulation; what is left of the cornea will clear up, and the eye get well. If the patient has any sight left, he is fortunate. Invariably the conjunctiva will be dragged into the cicatrices which the wounds leave.

Cause.—There is but one cause for diphtheritic conjunctivitis—direct infection by the Klebs-Loeffler bacillus.

The microbe must come in contact with the conjunctiva to excite the disease. The fact that diphtheria is so extremely common and the ophthalmia so rare is presumptive evidence that the conjunctiva is not at all susceptible. Many a physician has died of diphtheria contracted during the examination of a child's throat, the patient having coughed directly into the doctor's face. We know medical men do not, with their mouths open, examine diphtheritic patients, and very few protect their eyes with glasses. Yet, I can find but one recorded case of diphtheritic conjunctivitis con-

tracted in that way. It would seem that in some persons—very few—there is an idiosyncrasy favorable to
diphtheritic ophthalmia. What influence evil surroundings have over the susceptibility of the conjunctiva I am unable to say. Probably none, for the disease is no more frequent among the poor and neglected
than among the rich. The cases I have seen were adults,
living in well-ventilated houses on the open prairie.
They had no disease in the throat nor had they been
near diphtheria. It is unnecessary to again consider
the pathology of diphtheritic conjunctivitis; that has
been done in Chapter III.

Diagnosis.—The diagnosis is easy, although it may
be confounded with gonorrhœal ophthalmia, acute orbital cellulitis, phlegmon of the lids, and panophthal-
mitis. The similarity of croup and diphtheria in the
throat and larynx is not apparent in the eye.

Croupous and diphtheritic conjunctivitis are so
dissimilar that it is hardly necessary to differentiate
their characteristics. The appearance of the lids in
gonorrhœal ophthalmia and diphtheritic conjunctivitis
is much alike. In both the lids may be enormously
swollen. In gonorrhœa they are comparatively soft, in
diphtheria they are very hard. Disturbing the lids in
the first disease does not cause much pain; with care
they may be turned; in diphtheria the upper lid cannot
be everted without great suffering.

The discharge in gonorrhœal ophthalmia soon becomes purulent; in diphtheria the pus does not flow
until the disease has entered the second stage; then
there may be some excuse in mistaking them. Some
cases of orbital cellulitis, especially if the phlegmonous

inflammation has attacked the cellular tissue of the upper lid, may simulate diphtheria. But then there is always a certain amount of exophthalmos and there is no discharge of any moment. Both in that disease (orbital cellulitis) and diffused purulent choroiditis the œdema of the conjunctiva is so great that thickened folds of the mucous membrane project out between the lids. In diphtheria that never happens, unless by chance a perforating ulcer has opened the eye to septic infection.

Treatment.—In the acute stage of the disease it is impossible to make any treatment directly to the diphtheritic patch. All that can be done is to keep the eye as clean as possible; for which purpose nothing is better than hot injections of the bichloride of mercury 1:3000. It is best done by attaching a flattened hard-rubber tube to a fountain syringe. The object of making the tube flat is to allow it to slip easily under the lid. A glass tube heated in a flame until red, then compressed, will do equally as well. With such an instrument it is possible to reach the superior cul-de-sac and thoroughly disinfect the eye without hurting the patient too much. The object in the treatment is to prevent an extension of the false membrane and hasten the breaking down of that already formed. At the present time we are compelled to believe that injections of the diphtheria antitoxin are indicated. I have had no experience in that treatment of diphtheritic ophthalmia, but I think it will save the eye more certainly than any other. The lids should be covered with hot compresses, to hasten the advent of the purulent stage. From experience that has been found to be the quickest way to do it. But I think if the physician should see the case at the very beginning, ice-cold applications would be indicated. They would be good for the disease in all its stages if it were not that cold tends to inhibit the vital forces of the corneal tissues. There must be as much life there as possible to prevent the extension of ulcerative necrosis. Cold and hot applications, antiseptic washings, and the antitoxin injections are all any one can do. When the acute stage is passed and the blennorrhœa begins, the methods and means to control purulent ophthalmia are indicated.

The object is to save as much of the cornea as possible, with the hope that an artificial pupil may restore vision. The conjunctiva will be badly scarred, nothing can prevent it, nor can anything be done to remedy it until all signs of the inflammation are gone.

A doctor who saves an eye suffering from diphtheritic ophthalmia can congratulate himself on his good fortune and his ability.

CHAPTER XIII.

CONJUNCTiVITIS SCROFULOSA—PHLYCTENULAR CONJUNCTIVITIS.

A disease of the eye peculiar to children, characterized by a catarrhal inflammation of the conjunctiva, the development of one or more nodular infiltrates on the surface of the cornea or conjunctiva (phlyctenulæ), lachrymation, and intense photophobia. Strictly speaking, this affection may not properly belong to the conjunctival diseases, as it is more a corneal trouble. But since the authorities have always spoken of it as a form of conjunctivitis, it is not out of place in this book. If we believe that Bowman's membrane and the superimposed epithelium are a continuation of the conjunctiva over the cornea, we have reasons to think that in reality phlyctenular keratitis is a conjunctival disease, especially since we know that the eruption is not always limited to the cornea. At any rate, this classification is open to serious and interesting debate, which is out of place here.

The attack usually comes on at night. A child will awaken in the morning and complain that the light hurts its eyes. Little children will violently rub the eyes, cry, and bury the face in the pillow. Older children will say that there is something in the eye; they also avoid the bright light. When the mother tries to see what is the matter, she will find the child cannot open its lids, that there is a little swelling of the skin over the eye, and that there is an unusual flow of tears. The moment she takes the child up, it will hide its face on her shoulder. That alone is a characteristic symptom. A child with a foreign body under the lid will make a great fuss, but it will not seek the dark. If the nurse is an observing person, she may have noticed that for a day or so before the attack the child was a little restless, had not played around as usual, and that it had fingered its eyes. Such premonitory symptoms are not usually observed before, but remembered afterwards. From the beginning the symptoms increase in severity, the light becomes intolerable, the lids swell a little at the edges, and, if disturbed, are spasmodically shut. The excessive lachrymation scalds the skin of the cheeks, and the continual flow of the tears into the nose excites an inflammation of the skin around the nostril and of the upper lip. From that cause the child may have a lateral coryza. The patient refuses to eat and play, it sits in a dark corner of the room, with closed eyes and bowed head, or it will remain constantly on its mother's shoulder. As soon as the sun goes down, it brightens up, will open the lids a little, and take food.

If nothing is done for the child, it will do one of two things: either get well or get worse. It may lie around a few days, then open the eyes, and commence to play, and seem itself again. But the eyes do not look well and bright, there will remain a slight drooping of the lids. So it will go on for an indefinite time, when suddenly it will have another attack as bad if not worse than the first. When it does not by itself improve, the lids swell considerably, the irritation increases, and the

eczema about the nose, lips, and cheeks gets very bad.
Because of the lack of exercise and nourishment, the
child rapidly runs down. It will require so much continual attention that the entire household becomes exhausted and the patient a pitiable invalid.

What is it that has caused such a disturbance?
Probably nothing more than a little infiltrate on the
surface of the cornea, not larger than the head of a pin.
If the eye is now examined, which, by the bye, is very
difficult to do, it will be found that there is more or less
catarrh of the conjunctiva, and that the acute inflammation is limited to the anterior surface of the eyeball. At one particular zone of the cornea the conjunctiva will be very red and the blood-vessels enlarged.
Usually there is ciliary congestion all around the cornea, but about the inflamed spot the congestion is more
intense. Near or at the limbus of the cornea, towards the inflamed area, a little white spot may be
seen, prominent, well defined. This spot is at first an
infiltrate under the epithelial layer, but it soon breaks
down into an ulcer, which will have running towards it
a few parallel capillaries from the nearest edge of the
conjunctiva. The phlyctenule may be large and cres-
centic, its concave edge towards the corneal limbus.
Then there will always be found external to the infiltrate an ulcer connected to the conjunctiva by a band
of blood-vessels. It may be that two or more such
phlyctenules have coalesced, then the lesion is larger
and the vascular band broad and prominent. If the
conjunctiva is carefully examined, it is possible to find
similar infiltrates in it, and it is not unusual to see on
the inner surface of the lid, near its edge, a well-defined

ulcer.   Such are the usual appearances of an ordinary case.

The *pathology* of the disease is interesting.   Immediately under the epithelium of the cornea or conjunctiva collect a number of round cells which evidently are derived from the epithelium itself.   The massing of the cells elevates the epithelial layer and thus forms a nodule—a phlyctenule.   The lesion may appear at any part of the cornea, usually, however, about one or two millimeters from the limbus.   The cells may be absorbed.   As a rule, the bleb ruptures, leaving a superficial ulcer, which may heal without a scar, but usually the ulcer penetrates Bowman's membrane, and because the corneal stroma is then exposed, the ulcer becomes infected.   About this time a few blood-vessels shoot out from the nearest edge of the conjunctiva and reach the bed of the ulcer; soon the cells of the phlyctenule nearest the capillaries are absorbed, but the cells above the edge of the ulcer, remote from them—towards the center of the cornea—increase in number; the wall of the ulcer under them breaks down, and the capillaries follow along.   *In this way a little wave of ephithelial exudation passes over the surface of the cornea, leaving in its wake a narrow linear excavation filled in at the bottom with new blood-vessels.*

When such an ulcer heals it leaves a scar, which in young children may apparently disappear, but for a long time it can be seen by focal illumination.   The width of such an ulcer will correspond to the long diameter of the phlyctenule, but the ulcer through secondary infection may become inflammatory and spread laterally, then there is danger that it will penetrate the cornea. If it does, the moment the cornea ruptures the iris falls into the wound and heals there. That is a very unfortunate accident, for when the eye recovers, the entangled iris drags on the ciliary body, which in children often causes secondary glaucoma. There may be two or more phlyctenules on the cornea; some may coalesce, some will ulcerate, others will not; so it sometimes happens that the major part of the surface of the cornea—indeed, the whole—is covered by discrete and confluent patches of exudation and such a quantity of blood-vessels that there is a dense pannus, cutting off all view of the anterior chamber and iris. If the physician is not careful, he may make a mistake and believe that the keratitis is secondary to blennorrhœal conjunctivitis, especially since in these cases the catarrh will be so severe that the tarsal conjunctiva grows velvety. The history, the photophobia, and the lack of blennorrhœa should make a differential diagnosis easy. Not infrequently the disease attacks a trachomatous eye; then the diagnosis is very difficult. It is hardly necessary to remind the reader that conjunctivitis pustulosa and phlyctenular ophthalmia, although somewhat alike, are different diseases, and there should be no difficulty in recognizing them.

Cause.—For many years this disease has been called scrofulous ophthalmia. Perhaps this is a misnomer, for the bacteriologists have nearly convinced us that scrofula is a myth and tuberculosis a fact. It is true that the microscope and artificial cultivations do approach nearer exactness than any other of our methods of investigation. It is equally as true that there are

—10—

things we learn from clinical experience that cannot be
negatived by laboratory experiment.   The microscope
may tell us a cell is dead, or dying, but it cannot say
whether it is sick or well.

Until my faith was somewhat shattered by Koch's
investigations, I thought there was a condition of the
body, either inherited or acquired, wherein the cells of
the blood or connective tissue lost to some extent their
vital powers.   Such subjects would necessarily react badly to pernicious influences.   They suffered from
colds, catarrhs, diarrhœas, emaciation, and lymphatic
excitability.   Many of them were the offspring of
tuberculous parents.   They were light-haired, fair per
sons; often had bad teeth; rarely dull, usually pre-
cocious.   Such children we called scrofulous.   Some
thought they discovered a syphilitic ancestry, but now
it is proper to say "tuberculous."   It is not probable
that this condition is a constitutional stigmata of
degeneration?

Those who still believe in the scrofulous diathesis
may say that, often, phlyctenular conjunctivitis is a local reaction to an irritation in a scrofulous patient.   I
can assure them that this is a good foundation upon
which to base the treatment.   But it must not be forgotten that many children suffer from this disease who are
not scrofulous.   A very frequent cause is indigestion.
Nineteen times in twenty we will find that the children
of the well-to-do who suffer are those who are allowed
to eat everything and anything; candies, sweetmeats,
hot bread two or three times a day, apples and cakes in
the interim.   Babies fed on tea and coffee and enter-
tained by green bananas are the ones liable to this com-

plaint. Such pernicious dietary predisposes little children to attacks of ophthalmia, as it does to attacks of
dermatitis. Such are the constitutional causes. The
local causes are not known. It looks very much as if
a special microbe had something to do with it, for it is
significant that only local antiseptics will cure it. If
the illustration published by Fuchs in his text-book on

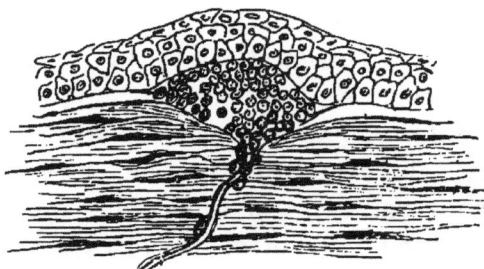

FIGURE 12.

The construction of a phlyctenule on the surface of the cornea, showing its
relation to a corneal nerve. (After Iwanoff.)

the diseases of the eye, taken from Iwanoff, is anatomically correct, it is possible that the nervous system has
something to do with it. In the drawing is shown,
where the phlyctenule rests on Bowman's membrane,
a corneal nerve penetrates the basement membrane
and is lost in the collection of new cells. This is significant, for it is possible that the phlyctenule is the result
of a nervous influence, as is the pustule in herpes
zoster. Some authorities teach that the eye-disease
is secondary to nasal disease; that the *materies morbi*
reaches the conjunctiva by way of the lachrymal duct.
Debilitated, scrofulous children nearly always have
some rhinitis, but there is no evidence that the ophthalmia is secondary, while there is proof that the trouble
in the nose comes directly from the irritation in the eye,

probably because of the constant flow of the tears into the nose, perhaps through the reflexis.

Diagnosis.—There should be no difficulty in recognizing this disease. The intense photophobia and lachrymation are suggestive, especially in little children. The white exudation on the cornea and the band of blood-vessels uniting it to the neighboring inflamed conjunctiva are characteristic. The little phlyctenules which suddenly come on the cornea in old cases of trachoma are somewhat similar to the phlyctenules in scrofulous ophthalmia, but anatomically there is no resemblance. Trachoma phlyctenules never appear in children; they rarely form in persons under twenty years of age, and then there are always marked evidences of degenerative trachoma—atrophy of the conjunctiva, scarred lids, etc. A foreign body may light upon and be rubbed into the cornea. If it is not removed, it will ulcerate off. Then there is some difficulty in determining the cause and character of the ulcer. Such ulcers may be quite large and yet there be no particular photophobia. The fear of light in scrofulous ophthalmia is not dependent upon the size or seat of the ulcer, but upon its peculiar character. Often on the upper limbus or edge of the cornea during the progressive stage of chronic blennorrhœal ophthalmia there will suddenly appear an irritable, ugly ulcer. If there is no pannus at the time, the blood-vessels will quickly shoot out towards it. These ulcers are very painful, the photophobia intense, and the lachrymation excessive. The beginner may mistake them for broken-down scrofulous phlyctenules. But in such cases there is always a history of chronic eye-disease and there are marked evidences of trachoma or blennorrhœa.

Phlyctenular conjunctivitis is sometimes seen in children about puberty and in young adults; it is then somewhat different in character from the disease in infants. There is not nearly so much photophobia, and very rarely, if ever, does the inflammation lead to the well-marked scrofulous pannus. Usually it is a simple corneal ulcer near the limbus, which has a tendency to inflame and break down. Such ulcers should not be mistaken for trachoma or blennorrhœal ulcers, nor the catarrhal ulcer in older people.

Colored people are often attacked by a peculiar form of conjunctivitis. The disease appears as a simple conjunctivitis, which is evidently secondary, for the characteristic lesions attack the conjunctiva of the eyeball. There is always ciliary congestion, which in black subjects, because of the pigmentation of the sclera, is difficult to see. At the extreme edge of the conjunctiva, on the corneal limbus, little round bead-like nodules appear. There may be a number of them, usually three; some are small, others large. The cornea is not often inflamed, but sometimes a little inflammatory ulcer will develop in the cornea adjoining the conjunctival growth. There is some photophobia, excessive lachrymation, no particular pain, but discomfort. Colored people of all grades and conditions are subject to it. But I have noticed that it is more common among the pure negroes. The disease is scrofulous ophthalmia.

Treatment.—The treatment is both constitutional and local, which must be combined in all cases. Both are extremely simple and satisfactory, for of all the

severe inflammations of the conjunctiva and cornea this
is the easiest to cure.   The first thing to do is to regulate the diet.   Hot bread, pancakes, tea and coffee,
and all other forms of indigestible food should be for-
bidden.   Let milk and water be the only drink.   Meat
once a day, chicken well cooked, and beef a little rare.
Pork, ham, and salted meats must be avoided.   The
ordinary vegetables will do no harm excepting, perhaps,
carrots and cabbage.   A little sugar is harmless, but
candy must be prohibited.   Cakes and sweetmeats
are bad.   It is better to let the child eat little and
often than to satisfy it at one meal.   Fresh air is as
necessary as good food.   The child must not be confined
to a hot, dark, ill-ventilated room.   If the photophobia
is so severe that it cannot go out, it is well to wrap a
handkerchief around its eyes and have it carried out.
It is imperative to give it the best possible hygienic
surroundings and by the improved dietary remove all
possible causes for reflex disturbances from the di-
gestive canal.   It is proper to prescribe a good emulsion of cod-liver oil, alone or compounded with the
hypo-phosphites.   They all demand some preparation
of iron.   From experience, I find that the syrup of the
iodide of iron is the best; twenty to thirty drops three
times a day, after meals, given in a little sugar or syrup.
The change of diet should correct any form of indigestion; if not, pepsin may help the stomach and small
doses of calomel regulate the bowels.   Such is the constitutional treatment.   It is rarely necessary to give
anodynes or opiates.   The local treatment is even more
simple, but it is essential that the physician should
know exactly the condition of the eye.   Sometimes

⌐ѕ.

that is very difficult to find out, for the examination of the eyes of these little patients is not easy. Because of the photophobia and the fear of the doctor, there is such violent spasm of the lids that they cannot be opened with the fingers wide enough to expose the cornea; lid-elevators are then necessary. I usually put a drop of cocaine between the lids. When ready, the child is held fast and steady by assistants. Then I open the lids with a spring speculum. If it is properly done, there is no danger of injuring the child. As soon as the lids open and the eye rolls up, I firmly grasp the conjunctiva below the cornea with a pair of forceps and pull the eye down. In this way one can see the character and extent of the disease. The spring speculum is not a good instrument to use if one feels he is not an expert; the ordinary lid-elevator will do, or one made by bending over the back of a hairpin. This operation should last but a moment. It is better to take a little time and see everything than to do it quickly and see nothing. Of course, the child will do a great deal of kicking and screaming; so if such disturbances are too much for the doctor and the parents, an anæsthetic is advisable.

Atropia is indicated in all cases, one grain to the ounce of water. One or two drops of this solution should be put into the eye three times a day. Nothing added to the atropia solution will add to its efficacy, unless it be a little cocaine. Morphine and astringents will do harm. All the preparations of mercury applied locally are specifics because they are powerful antiseptics. The ones usually selected are calomel and the yellow oxide. With a camel's-hair brush, a little dry calomel should be dusted on the conjunctiva of the lower lid once a day. Very little should be used, enough to be distinctly visible, as a powder on the mucous membrane. If a larger quantity is used or if it is lumpy, it will collect between the folds of the membrane and excoriate. The calomel is evidently changed by the fluids into the bichloride of mercury, and since it is not all acted on at once, but by degrees, it is evident that the eye is influenced for a longer time than it would be if a solution of corrosive sublimate were dropped in. The yellow oxide of mercury ointment, carefully prepared, 1 grain to the drachm of vaseline, is a popular remedy. Of this (golden ointment) a little piece is put under the upper lid once a day. When the photophobia is very severe and the child is suffering from spasm of the lids, I have found that the best remedy is an application of a mild solution of the nitrate of silver, 2 grains to the ounce. The inverted upper lid may be painted with this once a day, the excess washed off. This application will often act wonderfully; over and over again, I have seen children open their eyes twelve hours after it is used.

It is not well to try to relieve the blepharospasm by internal antispasmodics. They will do no good, but will irritate the stomach and counteract the improvements inaugurated by the new diet. Under this treatment the eye in mild cases should commence to improve in about four days. The local treatment must be continued until the child is well, the constitutional treatment longer. Some may be tempted to destroy the phlyctenule by the actual cautery. If one is proficient in handling that instrument, it may be tried, but it is rarely necessary; then again, it can do more harm than good. Whatever may be the condition of the cornea, atropia, calomel, or the yellow oxide are the best local remedies.

This is essentially a relapsing disease. Children rarely have but one attack; consequently it is advisable for the doctor to inform the parents of this fact and that there is danger of a relapse, especially if indiscretions in eating are permitted. As the child grows older the relapses become less frequent; finally cease.

It is to be regretted that scrofulous ophthalmia destroys many eyes, either through destruction of the cornea by ulceration, or because of secondary glaucoma caused by a bulging staphyloma holding in its cicatricial grasp the iris.

CHAPTER XIV.

—   —

XEROSIS,

The word "xerosis" is derived from the Greek adjective *xeros*, dry.   Xerophthalmia is a condition of the conjunctiva and cornea characterized by extreme dryness.   It is dependent upon one of two causes: either the mucous membrane is like an oiled surface and cannot be wetted, or there are no tears to moisten it.   In the chapter on the anatomy of the conjunctiva it was mentioned that the tears did not come alone from the lachrymal gland proper, but in part from the lachrymal glands under the upper lid and the minute racemose glands above the convex border of the upper tarsal cartilage.   From these two latter sources enough fluid can be secreted to keep the eye comfortable, for when the lachrymal gland is removed from the orbit, no bad effect is noticed other than that the individual cannot cry.   The tears are not only a solution of certain salts in water, but they contain some mucus and exfoliated epithelium.   The amount of the chloride of sodium in them is so great that they taste decidedly salty.   The object of the salt is to prevent the water swelling the epithelial cells, for when the epithelium covering the cornea is swollen or distorted, the acuity of vision falls.   Ordinarily the lachrymal flow is just sufficient to keep the surface of the conjunctiva and cornea moist.   The tears do not run over the eye, but are diffused over it by the action of the upper lid.

When the lid falls, it spreads over the eyeball the tears
that have accumulated above it; when it rises, it
spreads over the cornea and ocular conjunctiva an extremely thin layer of fluid from below, enough to soak
in between the superficial epithelial cells and by
osmosis replenish the water of the epithelial protoplasm lost by evaporation. If there are no tears or the
epithelium will not absorb them, the mucous membrane dries.

There are two kinds of xerosis, true and false.

False xerosis often occurs in exhaustive diseases
accompanied by coma—viz., typhoid and typhus fever.
chronic septicæmia, cholera, dysentery, and hysteria.
It is simply a drying of the conjunctiva, because there
are no tears and the patients lie for a long time with
the eyes open. The exposed epithelium of the cornea
and the conjunctiva becomes covered by a layer of
sticky mucus, which dries on the eyeball and along
the edge of the lids. The membrane immediately reacts
to the mechanical irritation; it becomes inflamed, so
there may be considerable redness and swelling. The
cornea clouds up, and, if not protected, may ulcerate.
Clinically this is a very serious condition, for the
majority of the patients die; yet the most marked case
I ever saw was a girl in hysterical coma. Her eyelids had not been closed for hours, so one can imagine
her condition. When she recovered, she had quite an
attack of conjunctivitis, but the cornea did not ulcerate.
The only treatment necessary in such cases is to keep
the eye moistened with salt water or glycerin and water and hold the lids shut by adhesive plaster. It is not
advisable to use a bandage for this purpose, for the

lids may open under compress and the cotton come in contact with the exposed cornea. This trouble never happens if there are any tears secreted; so long as the lachrymal glands functionate, the lids may remain opened indefinitely and the eye be kept moist, as is frequently observed in those with facial paralysis or deformity of the lids from burns.

Of xerosis proper there are two varieties; perenchymatous and epithelial. The first is quite common, the second very rare. One is dependent upon profound atrophic degeneration of the entire mucous membrane, the other upon disease of the epithelium. It is easy to understand how the conjunctiva can be totally destroyed by trachoma, chronic blennorrhœa, and ulcerative diseases. When a mucous membrane becomes transformed to a layer of dense cicatricial tissue, its function is abolished, and if it has any epithelium on it at all, it is deformed and useless. Such a condition of the mucous membrane is seen in pharyngitis sicca, atrophic rhinitis, and in old cases of granulated lids. In some the conjunctiva will be so shrunken that the cul-de-sacs are closed and the atrophied lids joined to the eyeball above and below the cornea like hinges. If the sensibility of the cornea is not benumbed by a pannus, there is no danger of xerosis, for the reflex action on the lachrymal gland is retained, and the tears will flow, although the ducts leading from the accessory glands are obliterated. In anæsthesia of the cornea the entire lachrymal apparatus may atrophy; then, of course, the dryness will be extreme and the mucous membrane changes to a layer of tissue resembling skin. If the student will notice the blind beggars on the streets, he will find some cases like these.

I do not know that anything can be done for advanced parenchymatous xerosis. If the case is seen in time, every energy should be exerted to retain the sensibility of the cornea and dissolve the pannus. For that purpose nothing can equal the sulphate of copper. A crayon should be slightly rubbed over the inner surface of the upper lid once a day. Massage with the yellow oxide of mercury ointment is good. When these do not arrest the progress, the case is hopeless.

The most remarkable of the different forms of xerosis is the epithelial. From some unknown cause the epithelium covering the ocular conjunctiva, especially that part most exposed to the air between the circumference of the cornea and the canthi, is altered in such a way that it will not absorb the water of the tears. Then, of course, the most superficial layers of the cells die. The patch has an opaque, frosty appearance, which makes it very prominent by comparison to the life-like surroundings. We do not know the changes that take place in the epithelial cells, but a particular bacillus has been discovered in the xerotic area, so, some believe it is dependent upon a local culture of micro-organisms. The probabilities are it is not a local disease, since nearly all the patients present other evidences of constitutional trouble; prominent among these is hemeralopia (night blindness); a defect of vision always a symptom of some intraocular disease, or the result of depressed nerve tone.

Xerosis epithelialis is seen in epidemics and among the poor and ill nourished. But people in the best of health may suffer from it, and it is not always accompanied by any visual disturbance. The epithelial cells evidently die and as foreign bodies excite a certain amount of inflammation. They are cast off or the patch sloughs away. In the first case new epithelium takes their place to live or die; in the second an ulcer is left to heal by granulation. Sometimes the disease attacks the cornea; then, if it leaves an ulcer, there is danger of the resulting leucoma interfering with vision. Usually little damage is done, for the disease disappears, either because it has run its course or the cause is removed.

The treatment should be constitutional and protective. Good food, cod-liver oil, and fresh air are requisite, and smoked glasses to protect the eyes from the glare of light, the dust, and the wind.

CHAPTER XV.

CONJUNCTIVITIS (HERPES, ACNE, ECZEMA).

In all diseases of the skin of the face there is a tendency to inflammation of the conjunctiva and cornea. The most common are herpes, acne, and eczema. Sometimes the inflammation passes from the integument to the mucous membrane of the eye; usually the disease attacks the conjunctiva directly, but at the time of the dermatitis. None of them (unless it be eczema) are dependent upon local irritation; they are constitutional eruptions. The ophthalmic surgeon is interested in three forms of herpes: herpes simplex, as it appears in herpes labialis, herpes zoster, and herpes iris. On very rare occasions a herpetic eruption appears on the conjunctiva of the eyeball and on the cornea. It comes suddenly and from the same causes that occasion its outbreak on the lips. This disease, when it attacks the eye, very closely resembles phlyctenular ophthalmia, but it is not apt to trouble children or young persons. The disease suddenly appears on the cornea as one or more minute blebs, which almost immediately rupture and leave small ulcers. The ulcers may be inflammatory—that is, infiltrated, or they can be so transparent that there is difficulty in seeing them, even under focal illumination. The accompanying conjunctivitis is always severe. There is a burning pain in the eye, great photophobia, and lachrymation. While some of the ulcers are healing, new vesicles may break out, but usually the first eruption is the acme of the attack and passes away in a few days. The ulcers are very superficial and leave but faint traces. Very few doctors will be on the look-out for this disease, so it is rarely diagnosticated correctly, unless the ophthalmia and dermatitis come simultaneously. The causes are the same that excite an outbreak of herpes around the mouth—viz., fever, indigestion, pneumonia, and menstrual disorders. The cases I have seen were women suffering from functional disorders of the reproductive organs; they all had such a history, and the monthly intervals between the attacks were suggestive. The treatment is very simple: solutions of atropia or eserine for the eye and proper medication for the body. The conjunctiva and the cornea will not stand anything but the most soothing applications. Astringents are contra-indicated, cocaine may moderate the pain some; atropia, a snug bandage, and warm applications are all that are necessary unless some complication arises.

In this place I shall call attention to a form of herpes which attacks the margin of the lids. In the intermarginal space, usually of the upper lid, where the ducts from the Meibomian glands open, one or more little blebs suddenly appear; they are transparent, being filled with an amber-colored fluid. The surrounding skin is not inflamed. On examination they look as if the ducts had become occluded and the blebs were the result. They are not connected with the ducts, for I have seen them between the mouths of the ducts and the lashes. The symptoms are simply annoying. The diseased spots may burn a little, but when the lids

come together in winking, they interfere, and worry the
eye like foreign bodies. They last from six to twelve
hours, rupture, then disappear. This is a very simple
affair, and all that is necessary to give immediate relief
is to puncture them with a needle. If the attacks are
frequent, it may be advisable to test the refraction and
prescribe appropriate glasses if they are indicated.

HERPES ZOSTER OPHTHALMICA.

This is one of the most painful diseases that can attack the eye. The cases are never mild, they are always severe. The trouble begins, like herpes zoster
in other regions of the body, with intense neuralgia and
hyperæsthesia of the skin; often it is over the distribution of the supraorbital nerve and the nasal branch of
the fifth; sometimes the pain is below the orbit in the
area supplied by the infraorbital nerve. The eye symptoms arise soon after the beginning of the neuralgia,
sometimes before the eruption on the skin. I can best
describe the disease by reporting the following case:

A gentleman twenty-five years old was suddenly
attacked by a most severe supraorbital neuralgia over
the right eye. The pain involved the same side of the
nose as far as the nostril. His doctor thought it was a
malarial attack and gave him large quantities of qui-
nine. The next day the eye was so congested that the
patient was turned over to me as an ophthalmic case.
On my first examination I could not tell what was
the matter, nor did I know for two days, when an eruption broke out over the brow and along the side of
the nose. The herpetic blebs reached the exact middle line of the face, and did not cross over to the other
—11—

side.   Seventy-two hours after the beginning of the pain a bleb appeared on the cornea, and with it came the photophobia and lachrymation.   The lesions on the skin suppurated, and, when they healed, left deep pits.   The bleb on the cornea broke down into an ulcer, which disappeared in a few days, leaving a scar. The subsequent effects were remarkable.   Soon after the eruption, the cornea became anæsthetized, which lasted several days.   There was marked paresis of the internal and superior recti muscles, which did not entirely disappear for months.   The iris, too, was paralyzed; the mydriasis remained half a year.   There was also developed an astigmatism, which still exists. For a long time I thought the astigmatism was lenticular, but now I am inclined to believe it is corneal, dependent upon the scar left by the lesion.   The particularly interesting clinical point in this case was the appearance of the conjunctivitis hours before the outbreak of the eruption either on the skin or the cornea.

Herpes zoster is a form of neuritis.   The skin over the area of distribution of the diseased nerve may be so low in vital tone that the ulcers left after the exfoliation of the scabs may become necrotic.   The same danger threatens the eye.   The corneal ulcers can enlarge and perforate the anterior chmber.   Such an accident I saw in an old man.   The cornea was almost destroyed by a secondary abscess.   The anæsthesia was so great that I had unusual difficulty in healing the wound after the abscess was incised and cleaned.

Diagnosis.—Until the eruption appears on the skin, it is not possible for the physician to make a correct diagnosis.   If the patient is subject to attacks of shingles, a sudden supraorbital neuralgia together with congestion of the eye may suggest herpes zoster. But that is unlikely, for few people have the disease a second time. The diseases of the eye somewhat like it in the beginning are iritis and glaucoma. There should be no difficulty in the differential diagnosis. In iritis the pupil is contracted and dilates slowly or irregularly under atropia, and there is always well-marked ciliary congestion. In acute inflammatory glaucoma the pupil is dilated, the cornea blurred and the eyeball very hard.

The cause of herpes zoster is not known. Most writers believe that it is of nervous origin; others think the inflammation is dependent upon disturbances of the circulation in the affected skin area. The bacteriologists see evidences of microbial invasion. I believe it is a neurosis.

The treatment is palliative; no internal or external medication will prevent the disease running its normal course. For the eruption simple drying powders are better than ointments or washes; for the eye atropia and a compress bandage are indicated. Since the corneal ulcer involves a tissue of low vitality, the physician should be careful not to further depress it, which will certainly happen if ice-cold applications are ordered, therefore, it is necessary to keep the eye warm. Nothing will surely relieve the pain but morphine. Cocaine is contra-indicated. If the coal tar preparations are used as analgesics, the physician must be careful, for only dangerous doses will be effective. The disease lasts from six to fourteen days.

HERPES IRIS OPHTHALMICA.

This is an extremely rare disease of the eye; very few cases have been seen or reported. The skin lesion is not more interesting to the dermatologist than the ophthalmia is to the oculist. The conjunctivitis is purely a croupous inflammation. The following translation of the report of a case by Von Arlt is an excellent description of the disease, although it is not as typical as the one I shall mention:

"A man fifty-seven years old was admitted to the clinic, suffering from inflammation of the eye, which was thought to be a conjunctivitis, for there was a gray deposit over the inner surface of the under lid. The conjunctiva of the retrotarsal folds was somewhat swollen, that covering the eyeball was not inflamed. It was the fifth day of the disease; evidently it was not diphtheria nor acute blennorrhœa. He had a herpetic eruption on the upper lip towards the angle of the mouth on the right side. It was very noticeable, but not carefully examined. After his admission on the eighth day, it was determined that it was not syphilis. At that time the inner surfaces of the upper and under lids were covered by a thin gray false membrane, which was quite adherent. Besides, he had an eruption over the palm of his right hand, which was recognized as herpes iris. The skin of the lids was somewhat red, but not swollen. The palpebral conjunctiva not covered by the membrane was thickly injected. The deposit extended from the folds to the edge of the lids, and was 0.5 m. thick; with forceps it could be torn away in shreds, would leave a bleeding spot, and soon re-form. The mouth became sore two days after the eye. A mottled gray-white membrane covered the greater part of the mucous membrane of the mouth. The upper and lower lips were covered by dried scabs. The inside of the cheeks, gums, hard palate, and sides of the tongue were covered by single and confluent patches of false membrane. Because of the pain in masticating and swallowing, the patient had eaten very little; in consequence, he was very much run down. The breath had the smell of fresh pus. During twenty-four hours the flow of saliva was 300—400 grams. It contained nothing abnormal. He had no disease in the throat, nose, or larynx. The disease of the skin appeared seven days after the disease of the eye; it began by an itching in the hand at night; the next morning there was a well-marked eruption over the palm. The young efflorescence was a hyperæmic spot about the size of a split pea, scarcely raised above the level of the skin, in its center was a dark red spot (a small hemorrhage). Shortly afterwards there appeared a red œdematous ring around the original patch, then another ring formed around it. When the efflorescence was completely developed, there were four concentric rings (two white and two red) around a central hemorrhage. The case progressed without fever. In two days, the membrane over the tarsal cartilage of the upper lid broke away, leaving exposed the reddened mucosa devoid of its epithelium. Nine days after he entered the hospital, the eye was free of false membrane. It left the conjunctiva slightly hyperæmic with some prominence of the papillæ. The eruption which appeared on the left palm, May 2d, showed the next day on the back of the right hand, then on the extensor sides of the elbows, finally on the soles of the feet and on the fingers of both hands; there, some were abortive, while others developed into large blisters filled with opaque serum. On the 27th of May the patient was discharged.

The following case I have reported once before. It is appropriate in this place, and, because it is so similar to the above, it is of particular interest.

In the spring of 1884, a lady, the mother of three children, the wife of a well-to-do farmer, was brought to me for treatment of her eyes. She was suffering from what appeared to be a complication of diseases. She was totally blind and had been so for one week. Two week before I saw her, she was taken ill with what was supposed to be an attack of indigestion. Her eyes inflamed a little, the lids closed and could not be opened; then an eruption appeared over the body and fever blisters on her lips. When I saw her, the condition was as follows: Over the legs and arms were scattered a number of round, well-defined, flat, hyperæmic patches. In the center of each was a dark red spot; some of the lesions were larger than others. A number of them had evidently disappeared, for they left dark blotches on the skin, which did not disappear on pressure. The palmar surfaces of her hands and the soles of her feet were covered by immense blisters, which were filled with serum. Her mouth was in a dreadful condition; both lips were covered by black hemorrhagic scabs, which extended up to the nose and down to the chin. Inside of the lips and cheeks was a dirty false membrane, tightly adherent. The mucous membrane of the fauces, tongue, and palate was not diseased. It looked like a very aggravated case of herpes labialis. The eyelids were closed; they were not swollen, and until they were separated no one would suspect that there was anything the matter with the eyes. When an attempt was made to part the lids, it was seen that they were closely adherent to a false membrane, which covered the eyeball. With care it was possible to peel the upper lid off the deposit. It left the mucous membrane raw, for it bled considerably. Nothing could be seen of the eye, for the croupous deposit evidently filled the entire conjunctival sac. With two pairs of forceps I gently tore a way through the membrane towards the cornea. When I had gone about one-eighth of an inch, I reached a space filled with clear fluid, which was in front of the cornea and showed that the deposit was not adherent to its epithelium. As soon as the opening admitted the light, the patient could see. There was no disease either of the cornea or deeper tissues. She did not suffer any pain about her eyes, she only complained that she could not open the lids. The treatment for the eyes was continued warm applications; nothing else was done. In a few hours the opening I made closed and the lids adhered again. There was no discharge. Gradually the membrane melted away. It got thinner and thinner and finally disappeared. When it was gone, I found it had completely stripped the epithelium off the conjunctiva and left it red, but not inflamed. The great difficulty, then, was to prevent the lids adhering to the eyeball. Every morning I was compelled to free them. The operations were painful and bloody. Oil and vaseline would not prevent the sticking together of the mu-

cous surfaces. The eyes got well, but the superior cul-
de-sacs were completely occluded. The skin disease
disappeared, the lips cleaned off, and the patient left
the hospital in six weeks.

ACNE CONJUNCTIVITIS.

If acne is an inflammation of the follicles and
glands of the skin dependent upon a local cause, it is
difficult to understand how the disease can attack the
conjunctiva and cornea, for it is very exceptional for
a dermatitis to encroach upon the mucous membrane lining the lids. People who have acne of the
face sometimes suffer from acute inflammation of
the eyes, and since it is more than a coincidence, the
authorities have described an acne ophthalmia. The
cause of the two diseases is evidently the same; therefore it is presumptive that certain forms of acne are
constitutional. The variety which interests the oculist is, acne rosea. That disease of the skin of the face
and nose is a familiar picture. The red skin, the swollen alæ of the nose, and the arborescent capillaries
shooting out from the naso-labial folds are characteristic. Scattered over the congested area are often
found little pimples, some tipped by a small pustule.
Such an affection we have always recognized as the
sign of high living, the mark of deranged digestion. It
is difficult to explain the relationship between the disease in the eye and that on the skin, for in this form of
conjunctivitis the skin lesion is not always prominent.
The worst cases are often in those who have no marked
acne of the face, but who suffer periodic attacks of
pimples.

Acne of the conjunctiva is very much like phlyctenular ophthalmia, inasmuch as there is a corneal
lesion—an ulcer—a certain amount of conjunctivitis
and the most intense photophobia. It differs from
scrofulous ophthalmia in two particulars: it does not
attack children and there are no capillary bands. The
ulcer is small, angry-looking, and persistent. It may
heal in a few days; as a rule, it will last for weeks. It is
essentially a relapsing disease; the second lesion
comes as the first goes. Although this disease is not at
all dangerous, so far as the eye is concerned, yet it is
very annoying. The photophobia may be so severe
that the patient must remain in a darkened room.

The best treatment is atropia, counter-irritation
over the forehead (the white precipitate ointment), and
tempered light. Brushing the inverted lids with a
mild solution of the nitrate of silver will sometimes
allay very much the fear of light and the blepharo-
spasm. Eserine has disappointed me in this, as it has
in other diseases of the cornea for which it has been extravagantly recommended. My experience is, that
destroying the ulcer with the actual cantery is the
best method devised to cut short the disease. Unfortunately, the ulcers are apt to come immediately in
front of the pupil; then the cautery is contra-indicated,
for the resulting scar will blur the vision.

The following case is a very good example of this
disease:

A lady forty years old was led into my office suffering with pain in the right eye and the most intense
photophobia. The eye could not be examined without
the aid of cocaine. When, by that means, the eyeball

was exposed, a small angry ulcer was seen at the upper
edge of the cornea.   There was considerable diffused
conjunctivitis.   It was the first time she had had anything the matter with her eyes. In hunting for the cause
of the ulcer, I found a few acne pimples scattered over
the cheeks and forehead. These she had not noticed, for
they evidently came out on the skin at the time the
eye was attacked.   Her general condition was good,
but she suffered considerably during her monthly pe-
riods.   I destroyed the corneal ulcer with the electric
cautery, put the eye under the influence of atropia, and
applied a compress bandage.   The relief was immediate, and in a few days the eye was well.   About three
months afterwards she had another attack in the same
eye, also an acne eruption on the face.   At that time
the ulcer was immediately in front of the pupil.   Fear-
ing the use of the cautery, I tried to heal the lesion by
atropia and bandaging.   They failed; escrine was substituted.   She then suffered dreadfully and could only
get relief from large doses of morphine.   I tried dubois-
ine, homatropine, and cocaine; was then compelled to
resort to the cautery; again she had immediate relief.
Six months after, she had another attack, with it the
acne.   But, as the eruption on the face was so decided,
I sent her to a dermatologist, who signally failed to cure
it. The corneal ulcer was extremely painful and in front
of the pupil. . Knowing that if the cautery were used,
she would never again have a useful eye, I declined to
operate.   She then went under the care of another
oculist. If I am to judge from the length of time she
wore a bandage, he had an experience similar to if not
worse than mine.

ECZEMA CONJUNCTIVITIS.

On rare occasions the irritative effects of eczema of the face extend to the eye, particularly so in eczema pustulosa and eczema capitis in children. It is doubtful if ever the characteristic eruption comes on the conjunctiva. Some cases have been reported in which, during the course of the skin inflammation, ulcers appeared on the cornea and the symptoms were very much like scrofulous ophthalmia. But it must be remembered that that is no proof the disease on the eye was like that on the skin, for it is not surprising for children with eczema about the head to have at the same time phlyctenular conjunctivitis. In adults it is different. When they, during the course of severe dermatitis of the face, suffer from subacute conjunctivitis together with circumscribed keratitis, it is presumptive that the same cause is inflaming the eye. In eczema of the face, with swelling of the eyelids, it is a rule to find a certain amount of conjunctivitis, but I do not know that I ever saw the cornea inflamed. It must be remembered that very often, when there is great photophobia and lachrymation, the eczema on the lips and cheeks is secondary, dependent entirely upon the tears moistening the skin. This is often seen in scrofulous ophthalmia.

Case.—A man was admitted into the Missouri Pacific Railway Hospital under the care of Dr. C. W. Davis, of this city, suffering from suppurative eczema of the face. There was considerable swelling of the skin; the eyelids were puffy and the conjunctiva very red. He complained that his eyes smarted and that the light hurt them. The conjunctiva was very much inflamed, but the cornea was clear. The conjunctivitis lasted until the face was well. It was not dependent upon a neighboring irritation, but had a constitutional cause.

PEMPHIGUS.

A very rare lesion of the conjunctiva associated with the disease of the skin is the pemphigus bleb. But few examples have been recorded. The majority of ophthalmic surgeons have never seen a case. It appears that the blister on the conjunctiva is exactly like that on the skin, but differs from it in one important respect: in the eye the lesion entirely destroys the mucous membrane under it; in the skin it does not. Consequently the results are exactly like those after diphtheria and burns: great shrinking of the conjunctiva and symblepharon.

CHAPTER XVI.

PTERYGIUM.

PINGUECULA.

To understand in part the etiology and nature of the pterygium, it is necessary to know something of an apparently harmless little growth in the conjunctiva next to the cornea, called the pinguecula. This can scarcely be called a disease, for the majority of adults in this section of the country have it. It is invariably seen on that part of the conjunctiva of the eyeball always exposed when the lids are open. Consequently, it may be on both sides of the cornea; usually it is only on the nasal side. To the reader it may be surprising to learn that nearly all men over thirty have pingueculæ. The reason why they are not generally noticeable is, they are often small and transparent.

The pinguecula is a little triangular growth in the conjunctiva on the nasal or temporal side of the cornea; its base on the circumference of the cornea, its apex toward the canthus. It appears to be a simple thickening of the membrane and does not encroach upon the transparent cornea unless it is subjected to continued irritation, when it is apt to grow towards the pupil and make the pterygium. The reason why so many people who live upon the Western plains have the pinguecula is, the eye is almost continually subjected to bright light, wind, and dust. Under these circumstances the people ride and go about with the eyelids almost closed to protect them; then the triangular area of the conjunctiva, which must be exposed that they may see, is alone irritated. When a mucous membrane is irritated, it does not, like the skin, protect itself by covering its surface with thick layers of epithelium; it simply hypertrophies. That is, there is an increase in the connective-tissue elements. So, in pinguecula the elastic fibers binding the conjunctiva to the sclera are greatly multiplied. Therefore the denser the tissue becomes the more anæmic it must be; so one can easily understand why in acute conjunctivitis the eyeball is deep red and the pinguecula pink. Most pingueculæ are white; many of them are amber color, because there is deposited in and between the connective tissue bundles of the tumor hyaline matter.

The growth is harmless and requires no treatment unless it crosses the edge of the cornea. Then it should be removed, which is best done by cocainizing the eye and dissecting off the tumor with a sharp, thin knife-blade; but care must be taken that all particles adhering to the sclera are scraped away. A stitch to bring the cut edges of the conjunctiva together is not always necessary.

THE PTERYGIUM.

A comet-like growth on the eyeball, its head on and adherent to the cornea, its tail radiating over the conjunctiva. It is very common in this country, especially among cattle-men. We see it and have an opportunity to study it nearly every day; yet of all the diseases of the conjunctiva this is under-

stood the least. It is nearly always on the nasal side
of the eye; rarely it is seen on the temporal side; then
there are two, an external and an internal, double
pterygia. Simply glancing at it, the pterygium looks
like a fleshy growth on the eye extending from the caruncle over into the transparent cornea. It is in the median line and on that part of the conjunctiva most exposed to the air. Sometimes it is fiery red and prominent; then it is very deforming. Unless inflamed, it is
rather transparent and not very noticeable, for the
majority of them are small. When the pterygium is
carefully examined, it will be observed, that if it is
large, most of the growth is below the exact horizontal
meridian of the eye, and that part on the cornea is a
distinct tumor, closely adherent and sharply defined
towards the pupil, to which a fold of the conjunctiva
is attached. It looks as if a growth started on the
white part of the eye, and, moving over the cornea,
dragged the mucous membrane with it. The neck,
that part which crosses the corneo-scleral line, is generally thick, and it is possible with a probe to find that
it is not flatly adherent to the eyeball, for there is usually a folding under of the conjunctiva above and below
it. It is distinctly striated and contains many parallel
blood-vessels. Starting at the neck, the tail gradually
spreads out towards the nose; it becomes very thin, and
may fade away entirely; it is fan-shaped. Because the
vessels and folds of the conjunctiva radiate towards
the neck, it looks somewhat like the wing of a fly, and
for that reason it is called pterygium. There are two
kinds of pterygia, true and false. A false pterygium
is nothing more than a duplication of the conjunctiva

adhering to the cornea. It results from ulcerative keratitis and shows that the cornea has been partly destroyed. When, in acute blennorrhœa, there is extreme chemosis and the surface of the conjunctiva is pushed into the bed of a corneal ulcer, it is possible for them to grow together; then, when the inflammation and swelling subside, the displaced fold of the conjunctiva remains attached. Such an accident can happen at any part of the circumference of the cornea; consequently such pterygia may be above or below the pupil and covered by the lids, which is never the case in the true variety. If the ulcer is exactly on the edge of the cornea, the resulting cicatrix may pull the conjunctiva over the scleral border; and, if a section of the cornea and conjunctiva are destroyed together, as in burns and diphtheria, the scar will always be a false pterygium.

One of the most interesting subjects in ophthalmic surgery is the nature and growth of the true pterygium. There are only two theories concerning it worthy of consideration, the Von Arlt and the Fuchs. Until the latter explained its development from the pinguecula, the accepted explanation was as follows: From some cause (usually an injury, often a disease), a small ulcer appears at the nasal or temporal side of the cornea exactly on the median line. The inflammation excited by the ulcer extends to the neighboring conjunctiva and causes a swelling of it. Because the chemosis is being continually compressed between the edges of the closing lids, its epithelial surface is forced against the bed of the ulcer and becomes fixed by inflammatory exudation, exactly as was described the formation of false pterygium. Of course, the fold of the mucous membrane

will be considerably elevated above the surface of the
cornea, and, at the edge of the ulcer, towards the pupil,
will be sharp and steep. In the healing process the corneal and the conjunctival epithelium do not fill in the
angle, and because that little linear pocket is irritated
by foreign substances, catarrhal secretion, wind, etc.,
the ulcer remains. The irritation being continued, the
inflamed head of the pterygium follows the ulcer as it
moves towards the center of the cornea. During this
time, inflammatory products are added to the tissues
making the head of the growth. As the new connective tissue grows, the old cicatrizes, and will either
tear the tumor off the cornea or pull the conjunctiva
to it. The latter usually happens, for the mucous membrane is loose and elastic, whilst the attachment to the
cornea is strong. In this way the tumor advances
towards the pupil. So long as the ulcer is present and
the head inflamed, the pterygium is progressive.

If the ulcer heals, the growing process stops, the
inflammation subsides, and the head atrophies, but the
nodular cicatrix remains. Now comes the ingenious
reasoning why the pterygium does not go beyond the
center of the cornea, for it is evident that, if the ulcer
does not heal, the growth will cross to the opposite side.
Von Arlt is silent on this point, but Fuchs well explains it. The cornea receives its nourishment from the
vessels of the conjunctiva and episcleral tissues surrounding it, whose capillaries terminate just inside of
the transparent membrane. The nutrient fluids are
thrown off from this circular band and flow towards the
center of the cornea. When the pterygium crosses the

—12—

scleral line and becomes fixed to the underlying tissues by inflammatory exudate, it constricts or oblit-
erates the blood-vessels under it; consequently, that
segment of the cornea receives less nourishment than
its surroundings, but it is well supplied from the
lymphatic channels at its sides. Now it is evident
that the circulation of the lymph is greater near the
edge of the cornea than at its center, so as the head advances towards the pupil it gets into the region of least
vitality, when the amount of inflammatory material
thrown off becomes less and less, until there is not
enough to drag the steep wall of the conjunctiva down
to the level of the ulcer. The head of the pterygium
ceases to be irritated; the inflammation subsides and
the ulcer has a chance to heal. Again, the further the
head is from the edge of the cornea the greater the
tension of the tail; so when the pull of the conjunctiva
equalizes the drag of the cicatrix at the head, the
growth can advance no further. For that reason, a
pterygium with a narrow head will not go very far; a
broad one may reach the center of the cornea. This explanation accounts for the development of the pterygium, but a serious objection to it is, there is not always
a progressive ulcer piloting the head. This is easily
overcome. It takes from five to fifteen years for a
pterygium to advance over the cornea one-fourth of an
inch. It is certain that an irritable ulcer would reach
the pupil in a few weeks. If the theory is correct, it is
evident that at the head of the pterygium there is very
seldom an ulcer; so one rarely has an opportunity to see
it. In fact, the growth advances a little at a time and
at very long intervals; consequently it may be said they

are all progressive, but for months and months stationary. It is not necessary that the ulcer should extend below Bowman's membrane. At the angle there may be simply an epithelial defect which allows the two basement membranes to come together and adhere, as we have seen they will do in the chapter on croupous ophthalmia. Pterygia of this kind are loosely attached to the cornea and easily pulled off.

Very often the pterygium develops from the pinguecula, as Fuchs has very well explained (Graefe's "Archives," 1892, Part 3). In these instances the tumor advances from its seat on the sclera over into the cornea and pulls the conjunctiva with it. The head is not led by an ulcer, for the growth does not always move over the surface of the cornea, but under it. The pinguecula is a connective-tissue tumor, and enlarges at its periphery. Why it should grow towards the center of the cornea is not known. Possibly it is, that that part of the cornea immediately in front of the tumor is the place of least physiological resistance because of the embarrassed circulation. The advancing edge of the growth pushes along under Bowman's membrane between the superficial layers of the cornea, and it has in front of it a zone of keratitis, which can be distinctly seen through a lens. These pterygia are always progressive; it is only a question of time when they will reach the pupil.

Since the neck and tail are made up of folds of the conjunctiva, they sometimes develop cysts, because two adjoining surfaces unite and close in a pocket of the mucous membrane. Such a cyst I have removed as large as a pea.

I believe there are two kinds of true pterygia; that Von Arlt was correct, Fuchs also.

Beyond the disfiguration, pterygia are harmless, unless they encroach upon the area of the pupil. Then they interfere with vision. Not alone will the head cut off the rays of light, but it will disturb the refraction and curvature of the cornea a considerable distance beyond it; so we may find with a small tumor annoying disturbances of vision. They are easily inflamed, then they become very red and irritable, and their presence alone may excite chronic conjunctivitis. Very large pterygia hinder the free outward rotation of the eye, which is often distressing.

Treatment.—There is but one thing to do—remove the tumor. Anything else is not even palliative. The nitrate of silver, calomel, tincture of opium, etc., will do no good. The pterygium must be cut away, and the sooner it is done the better. There are many ways to do it; the best is to cut the head off from the surface of the cornea, which permits the tumor to shrink towards the canthus. If it does no do so sufficiently, help it by snipping the conjunctiva with scissors. Then with a sharp knife scrape the shreds and remnants off the sclera and cornea. With one or two stitches bring the conjunctiva from above and below and cover as much of the wound as possible. This is the ideal operation, and all other plastic methods are modifications of it. If it is successfully done, the true pterygium will not return, but the wound may, and very often does, suppurate; then, since it must heal by granulation, there is a scar left, which makes the false pterygium. This is a

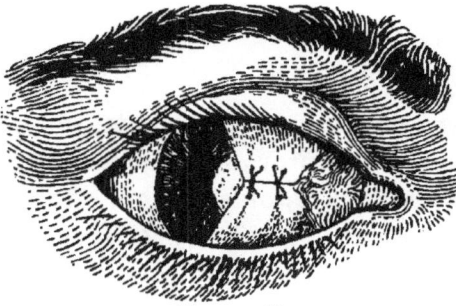

FIGURE 13.
Operation for pterygium, completed.

deforming as the true, but it will not advance. It is for
this reason the operation is often, apparently, unsuc-
cessful. Now, the smaller the wound the greater the
hope that it will heal by first intention; consequently
the smallest pterygium should be removed, and if a
pinguecula crosses the edge of the cornea, it calls for an
operation. When the head of a pterygium encroaches
upon the pupil, very little is to be gained, so far as the
vision is concerned, from the operation. If the patient
is quite blind, it is best to leave the tumor alone, but
make an iridectomy upwards.

CHAPTER XVII.

TUBERCULOSIS OF THE CONJUNCTIVA.

When we consider the universal distribution of tuberculosis and the prevalence in the atmosphere of Koch's bacillus, it is astonishing that tubercular conjunctivitis is so rare. I have never seen a case which was proved to be tubercular by bacterial investigation, although I have seen some, in my own practice, which I thought were tubercular. The probabilities were that I was mistaken. Anyone who is familiar with the disease in the pharynx and understands the pathological anatomy of tubercular growths can picture the disease as it affects the conjunctiva.

From physical and histological causes, primary tuberculosis of the conjunctiva selects two parts of the membrane in preference to any other—the superior retrotarsal folds and the conjunctiva of the upper lid a little internal to its edge, where foreign bodies are most frequently found. This is evident, for in these two localities the tubercle bacillus has a chance to remain long enough to implant itself. In some respects the disease resembles trachoma, for the membrane is covered with granulations, which may project in masses down from above. The lids are thick and heavy, the entire mucous membrane swollen. If any of the tubercular surface is ulcerated, there will be a purulent discharge very much like that in blennorrhœa. In an eye in this condition one would expect the cornea to be-

come involved; consequently there is either irritative
or ulcerative pannus, for it is only a matter of time
when the disease attacks the conjunctiva on the eyeball. Then, as in trachoma, the infiltrate rapidly
breaks down. An ulcer, once started at the edge of the
cornea, will soon reach the anterior chamber and open
the interior of the eye to tubercular invasion. In the
majority of cases the lymphatic glands connected with
the diseased eye are infected, and it will be observed
that the lachrymal sac is often filled with granulations,
but this is not peculiar to tubercular conjunctivitis, for
it is seen in trachoma.

We know that the conjunctiva is very rarely
attacked by the tubercle bacillus; consequently the
disease is in the nature of an accident; so for the two
eyes to become infected at the same time is an improbable coincidence, but it is not impossible. The only
disease it can be mistaken for is trachoma, but if the
reader will compare the histories and pictures of the
two, and remember that trachoma of such severity
would never be confined to one eye, the differential
diagnosis should be easy. Should the physician see a
case which he thinks is tubercular, unless the bacillus
is found in the discharge, it is better for all concerned
to believe himself mistaken, and to make the diagnosis
by exclusion, for the granulations coming from an old
chalazion, and the granulations which collect about a
foreign body buried in the tissues of the upper cul-de-
sac may deceive him. An ulcerating gumma or an
epithelioma of the conjunctiva can worry the diagnostician not a little.

In both these there may be adenitis of the preauricular ganglion. Indeed, the lymphatics can be swollen in all suppurative diseases of the conjunctiva, especially if there are ulcers admitting to the deep tissues the septic microbes. Tubercular conjunctivitis is a malignant disease. The focus must be removed, even if it is necessary to destroy the eye. When the diagnosis is confirmed by the microscope or tuberculin injections, the sharp curette should be used and the wound dressed in iodoform.

LUPUS.

It is well determined now that lupus is a form of tuberculosis, for the Koch bacillus is found in the indurated tissues about the ulcer. Lupus of the conjunctiva is usually an extension of the disease from the skin of the lids, although cases of primary lupus conjunctivitis have been reported. In these Western States lupus of any kind is comparatively rare. In those countries where the disease is common lupus of the conjunctiva is seldom seen. The disease may be mistaken for epithelioma, and, unless one has had considerable experience in skin diseases, the differential diagnosis cannot be made without the aid of the microscope. The treatment is the same as in tubercular conjunctivitis, but it is not necessary to be so heroic. The disease is essentially chronic, and there is no danger of systemic infection.

CHAPTER XVIII.

SYPHILIS OF THE CONJUNCTIVA.

When the close relationship between the mucous membrane of the eye and the skin is considered, it is not surprising to learn that syphilitic diseases of the conjunctiva are not uncommon. The reason why they are not oftener seen is, they are not looked for, unless there is a deformity or the patient directs the attention to the eye. If the physician will examine through a glass the conjunctivæ of all persons suffering from secondary syphilis, he may be surprised to find that often the eruption is nearly as distinct there as on the body, especially if the dermatitis is of the erythematous variety. For that reason the text-book authorities write of the intractable conjunctivitis of syphilis. There is always a cause for conjunctivitis. As in some of the exanthematous fevers (measles, for example) the conjunctiva and the skin react to the same poison, so in syphilis.

The conjunctiva is subject to chancre, macular and papular eruptions, gumma, mucous patches, and ulcers. Hunterian chancre of the conjunctiva is comparatively a rare lesion; few cases are reported; but it is much more common than is generally supposed. The spot of inoculation appears on the inner surface of the lids near the edge or at the cul-de-sac. Chancre in these places behaves exactly as it does on the penis. There is great swelling, painless induration, and enlargement of

the lymphatic glands of the head and neck, especially
the preauricular gland.   However severe the lesion
may be, there is little danger that it will leave a deforming cicatrix, unless it is badly treated or it is placed
on the eyeball. Such a case was reported by Mackenzie.
The inoculation usually happens by infecting the eye
from the mouth—kissing the eyelids. The disgusting
habit common among some people of cleaning the eye
of foreign bodies by the tongue has been responsible
for many of these cases. The diagnosis is easy; there
is nothing I know of like it.   Epithelioma can be ex-
cluded by the history and the course. Certainly no
careful doctor ought to mistake a chancre for a chalazion; yet I know that has happened. The treatment
is scrupulous local cleanliness, mercurial inunctions,
and dusting the chancre with a little dry calomel once
a day.

Mucous patches on the conjunctiva are rare lesions.
They look like mucous patches elsewhere; they appear
most frequently on the extreme inner edge of the lids
and on the outer half of the lower cul-de-sac, but they
have been seen near the nose. They heal readily on
internal and local treatment, but they may ulcerate and
act badly, which is undoubtedly the reason why the
older authorities wrote so freely of syphilitic ulceration
of the conjunctiva and lids.

I have seen two cases of gumma of the conjunctiva, more correctly gumma under the conjunctiva, but
involving the membrane. In both the mucosa of the
eyeball was affected.   In one, the tumor was very
much like an aggravated episcleritis; at the same time

there was a gumma in the iris. They improved rapidly
on mixed treatment. These tumors may break down
and ulcerate, when it will be a hard task to differentiate between them and certain malignant diseases;
epithelioma, for example. But if the reader will not
forget that all suspicious tumors about the eye, especially in young persons, demand a course of the
iodide of potash preliminary to operative interference,
there will be little danger of a mistake. Either because we are gradually becoming immuned or our
treatment is greatly improved over that of Mackenzie's
time (1854), destructive syphilitic disease of the conjunctiva and lids is almost unknown. Certainly no
modern author could report such a list as that writer
did in his text-book of the diseases of the eye.

CHAPTER XIX.

TUMORS OF THE CONJUNCTIVA.

It is not intended to consider in this chapter benign or malignant diseases of the conjunctiva, which have encroached upon it from the surrounding tissues. I shall only mention those diseases which can and do primarily attack the mucous membrane, and from that focus extend indefinitely. Many of these tumors are very uncommon, but the subject is so important and interesting that it demands more than a passing notice.

Tumors of the conjunctiva are benign and malignant; some of them are connective-tissue growths, others epithelial; some start from blood-vessels, others from the lymphatics. No part of the conjunctiva is exempt, but where the membrane crosses the edge of the sclera to cover the cornea is the favored seat for their development, especially if they are malignant. Many tumors of the conjunctiva are congenital; the majority are acquired.

Simple granulation tumors (proud flesh) start from a granulating wound or from the edge of a fistulous opening. They frequently follow operations for squint. A chalazion which has ruptured through the mucous side of the lid will always have granulations around the opening, and because from the pressure of the eyeball the granulations are flattened out over an indurated area in the lid, they may look malignant. A probe and sharp curette will quickly clear up the diagnosis. A mass of exuberant granulations projecting down from the upper cul-de-sac behind the lid is a certain sign that there is a foreign body buried somewhere in the tissues or a pus cavity is in communication with the conjunctival sac.

I was talking one afternoon with Prof. R. Berlin (Stuttgart), when a young girl came into his office with a monocular blennorrhœa. When he turned the upper lid, a quantity of granulations sprang forward from above. Without asking a question, he reached for a pair of forceps, and, pushing through the mass of proud flesh, caught and pulled from the orbit a splinter of wood an inch and a half long. We were all astonished but him. Experience had taught him that that condition was usually caused by a foreign body.

Granulating tumors may be excited to grow by continued irritation. A tight, ill-fitting, rough artificial eye will do it, especially if the individual sleep with the eye in. When an eye is removed and the wound allowed to heal under a clot, the edges of the conjunctiva and the tissues around the head of the nerve come together and a little granulating tumor will grow. At first it is quite broad, but when the healing tissues constrict its base, it is transformed to a polypus. Until the tumor is removed, the stump will suppurate. It can be cut away with a pair of scissors sharply curved on the flat. The best way to remove a quantity of granulations is to scrape them off with a sharp spoon. If the surgeon attempts to remove them with scissors and does not cut them all off with one snip, the bleeding will embarrass him and he may injure the eye. Unless the cause is removed, they will return. Chal-

azions must be cleaned out and foreign bodies taken
away.   It would be quite an extensive and painful
operation to scrape off a large quantity of proud flesh
caused by an artificial eye.   It is better to cut away as
many as possible with scissors and reduce the rest by
applications of the nitrate of silver, 10 to 20 grains to
the ounce.   In doing this great care must be taken that
the caustic does not come in contact with the healthy
membrane, or cicatrices may be formed which will prevent the wearing again of the false eye.

WARTS (PAPILLOMA).

The common warts found on the skin sometimes
grow on the conjunctiva, where they may be seen
scattered over the lower cul-de-sac and grouped about
the caruncle.   They are never very large; sometimes
they look like little condylomata; usually they are papillary.   These growths are soft, but do not bleed when
disturbed.   They do not directly cause any irritation, nor can it be asserted that they are produced by it.
Sometimes they will interfere with the fitting of the
lower lid to the eyeball; consequently the eyes may
be suffused with tears.   I have never seen them in
adults; my patients were always young.   In my cases
both eyes were affected.   I could not discover the
cause, but I am inclined to the opinion that warts,
both on the skin and mucous membrane, result from
a local irritant, perhaps mechanical or chemical, probably microbic.   I once saw a papilloma spring from
the mucous edge of the lower lid below the caruncle.
When the lids were closed, it projected forward and was
exposed at the internal canthus.   The patient was a

young boy, 14 years old. The tumor was removed three times. I finally stopped its return by touching its base with the actual cautery.

It is a difficult thing to remove warts from the skin; it is harder to cure them when they attack the conjunctiva. We cannot destroy them by touching them with caustics or dusting them with calomel; they must be removed, and if they are grouped about the semilunar fold and caruncle, it is much easier said than done. The cases I have had were cured after months and months of careful attention. Each individual wart was cut off the conjunctiva and its base immediately cauterized with a red-hot platinum point. If the reader ever has a case—the patient, a nervous child —he will have cause to appreciate the difficulties I have mentioned. When operative interference is impossible, it is advisable to treat them on antiseptic principles. One or two drops of a solution of the bichloride of mercury 1 to 2000 should be put in the eye in the morning, and a mild astringent collyrium used at night. The sulphate or acetate of zinc or the acetate of lead in solutions of appropriate strength are serviceable.

FIBROMA.

The basement substance of conjunctival warts and papillary growths is composed of fibroid tissue, which is limited in quantity. If, however, it should be more diffused, making what is generally called a tumor, the growth is a fibroma. Excepting pingueculæ and pterygia, fibroid tumors of the conjunctiva are very rare; then they are either congenital or reach the mucous membrane from the deeper tissues.

The following case is interesting on clinical grounds, for it was probably diffused myxofibroma of the conjunctiva. I am not certain, however, for I did not have an opportunity to examine it microscopically.

A young lady, 22 years old, consulted me for disease of her eyes. Some years before she noticed that yellow spots appeared on her eyeballs; that they gradually grew larger, and, coalescing, covered the white of both eyes. She had no pain; could see very well, but the deformity distressed her. The eyeballs up to and all around the cornea were covered by a semitransparent yellowish membrane. It looked exactly as if a pinguecula had grown and involved the entire ocular conjunctiva. It was composed of a number of flat tumors. Around the cornea they were hard and quite thick, 1.5 millimeters or more, but towards the equator they became smaller, thinner, and gradually faded away. The tissue was too opaque to see the underlying vessels, nor was it itself well supplied with blood. That part of the conjunctiva involved was adherent to the episcleral tissues; consequently it could not be moved over the sclera. The thickened tissues were not very hard; they could be easily indentated by a probe. The cornea were clear; there was no discharge or evidences of inflammation. Both eyes were exactly alike. I could not remove the growths, but, believing that if small areas of the tumors were violently inflamed, they might be absorbed, I caught parts of the tumor between the blades of forceps and crushed them. In that way much of the deformity was removed. My diagnosis was, myxofibro-matous disease of the conjunctiva.

Fibroid tumors involving the conjunctiva from within the orbit are very deceiving, for they are much larger than they appear. The physician may start to cut away what he thinks to be a little tumor, and find before he is through that the supposed little affair extends into the depths of the orbit.

Lipoma (fatty fibroma) are more common, but it must be remembered that in the cases reported the disease started either in the subconjunctival tissue or in the orbital cellular tissue. They are congenital, and are found principally on the upper outer part of the eye, between the superior and external recti muscles.

CYSTS.

Small retention cysts are quite common; they often grow from the neck of a pterygium, starting from a pocket of mucous membrane caught between the folds of the conjunctiva. Some may develop into tumors as large as a pea. Most of them are small.

Dermoid cysts are, of course, congenital. Such cysts of the conjunctiva are on the eyeball near the cornea, and may contain growing hairs. We should not forget that a transplanted cilium from a trauma of the lids may develop a cyst under the conjunctiva. I have seen several dermoid cysts of the conjunctiva and cornea. They were in children, and could not be removed without endangering the eye; consequently they were let alone, especially since they were in babes and did not seem to be growing. It is doubtful if cysticercus cysts ever develop in the conjunctiva; usually

—13—

under it. Then, again, they are so extraordinarily rare that the subject needs no further comment.

SARCOMA.

Not an infrequent tumor of the conjuctiva is the sarcoma, which may be white or melanotic. The favorite seat for them is over the corneo-scleral junction and the caruncle, although these growths can appear at any part of the mucous membrane. They look like small fleshy tumors, round, flat, lobulated, or papillary. Some bleed, others do not. As a rule, these tumors spring from the episcleral tissue; many of them are pigmented and start from congenital moles of the conjunctiva. They are usually malignant, but not so much so as we have been taught to believe. There is a vast difference between the malignancy of an intraocular melanosarcoma and a pigment tumor of the conjunctiva: so much so that some are inclined to the opinion that many melanotic tumors of the conjunctiva may be benign. This opinion is not based on the text-books, but on the fact that so many of these tumors have been removed without a return, which is not the history of black sarcomas elsewhere. I once removed an inky-black tumor from the orbit of a woman who had had her eye enucleated some years before for disease. The growth was about the size of a large marble, and was surrounded by a dense white capsule. It did not, to my knowledge, return, for she is still living. I attended her about ten years ago. Dr. Sattler, of Cincinnati, has had considerable experience in conjunctival and subconjunctival melanomas; he, too, believes in the benign character of some of these growths. Sarcoma of the conjunctiva attacks principally adults. In making a diagnosis of these tumors the physician should distinguish between a primary and a secondary tumor, for not infrequently a sarcoma of the choroid perforates the sclera and appears as a black swelling under the conjunctiva, projecting up from the depths of the orbit and from the interior of the eye. Such eyes, of course, are blind. Then the prognosis is very bad; all the soft structures in the orbit must be removed, even the periosteum.

Sarcomas of the conjunctiva must be completely removed. Many of them simply cover the cornea, and can be cut away without destroying the eye. Diffused melanoma of the palpebral conjunctiva is a very difficult disease to deal with. It should be removed and the defect covered by a skin- or mucus-graft. We always hear of these operations when they are successful, but, unfortunately, the failures are lost to ophthalmic literature. ·

CARCINOMA.

True cancers of the conjunctiva are rare; most of them start at the edge of the lids, at the internal canthus and involve the mucous membrane secondarily. Carcinoma may appear at the caruncle, when it is especially dangerous and difficult to cure. Epithelioma of the conjunctiva proper nearly always comes on the eyeball and springs from the corneal edge of the membrane. I have a very beautiful specimen of a carcinoma I removed from the conjunctiva midway between the cornea and the external canthus, about over the insertion of the external rectus muscle. It was in the conjunctiva, and was removed without any difficulty. It did not return. The tumor was about the size and shape of a split pea, white, and as hard as cartilage. Under the microscope it proved to be an epithelioma. The further a cancer is away from the internal canthus the better the prognosis. In all cases it should be removed, even if the eye is sacrificed. Cancer of the caruncle is very bad, for however heroically it may be cut away, there is danger of a fatal return. The great trouble is, until a cancer about the eye ulcerates, there is no certainty in the diagnosis. It is very well to be wise when we have a nicely stained section of a tumor under the microscope, but we must remember that we cannot slice off a piece from a man's eye as easily as from his turbinated bones; consequently there is always danger that the neoplasm will get a good start before we are prepared to operate. Suspicious growths on and about the eyes should be first subjected to anti-syphilitic treatment for a time; then, if necessary, removed. It is better to lose an eye, even both, than die of cancer of the face.

ANGIOMA.

Angioma of the conjunctiva are rare tumors. I have seen them under the mucous membrane, but never in it. Wine-marks of the skin of the face and eyelids do not, as a rule, encroach upon the conjunctiva; such a case would be an interesting curiosity. There is nothing to be done for them. Wine-marks on the skin may be removed and the defect covered by a skin-graft; that could not be done on the eye.

Not infrequently in old people little calcareous deposits form in the Meibomian glands. They soon irritate the eye as foreign bodies. They can be removed by a flat needle.

CHAPTER XX.

WOUNDS AND INJURIES OF THE CONJUNCTIVA.

FOREIGN BODIES.

The most common accident is the reception into the conjunctival sac of a foreign body. Very few writers give the subject more than a passing notice; yet, of all the injuries to which the eye is liable, these are the most important, because of their frequency and the distress and annoyance they often give the patient. Foreign bodies are of all sizes, shapes, and grades—coal-cinders, sand, vegetable matter, pieces of stick, eye-lashes, bugs, insects, etc. I have removed worms from the conjunctival sac, and I have known a bug to set up such a dreadful inflammation with sloughing of the conjunctiva that it was almost impossible to tell whether the trouble was a trauma or a disease. Again, I have seen the eye badly mutilated in an attempt to remove what was thought to be a cinder on the cornea, but what was in reality a pigment speck on the iris.

The majority of small pieces of stone and cinder which alight upon the conjunctiva and cornea are wiped off by the lids or washed away by the tears; they pass along the border of the lower lid, reach the internal canthus, and leave the eye at the nose. But it depends largely upon the force with which the foreign body strikes the eye whether it can be thus removed;

then again, the size of the object is material. A large
hot cinder may strike the cornea with great force, as
often happens when one thrusts his head out of a car
window and looks toward the engine. The cinder
glances or rebounds off the eyeball, or is caught between the closing lids. If the body is small, it may
stick to the epithelium, and when the lid comes down,
pass under it. Ninety-nine times in a hundred the
individual immediately rubs his eye; this forces it
deeper into the cornea or into the conjunctiva of the
upper lid. Then the tears flow, and may wash it
away. Sometimes they fail to do so, when it must be
removed or work its way off. A small body on the
conjunctiva or cornea may let the lid pass over it and
be caught in the little depression behind the epithelial
cushion at the mucous edge of the lid as the lid rises
again. That is the reason why so many little cinders
are found adhering to the bottom of the upper lid.
Often a foreign body buries itself deep in the membrane or cornea, which happens in blasting accidents or
premature powder explosions. In the first the flying
stones usually destroy the eye. When it is spared, the
conjunctiva is badly lacerated. In gunpowder injuries
the conjunctiva is generally dotted over with half-burnt
powder-grains, which usually enter in and under the
membrana propria. If the face is very near the explosion, the cornea and conjunctiva may be badly
burnt. The condition of the lashes and eyebrows is a
good indication of the nearness of the fire.

In large manufacturing towns injury of the eye
from emery-dust is very frequent. It happens in

sharpening edged tools. The small particles of stone
or steel fly with great rapidity, and, when they strike
the eye, bury themselves. They have no deleterious influence on the conjunctiva, but they are extremely irritating to the cornea. When small splinters of wood,
straw, twigs—indeed, anything long and narrow—get
well up under the upper lid, they are apt to lodge in
the upper cul-de-sac, where they remain and set up considerable irritation. Then there is usually a purulent
discharge. If the foreign body wounds the conjunctiva
and is half-buried under that membrane, it will certainly start the growth of granulations (proud flesh).

Most insects contain formic acid. When they strike
the eye and get caught under the lid, they are generally
mashed during the first rubbing; the acid reaches the
eye and causes an intense burning, which usually lasts
a minute or so. Although bugs have legs, sharp-pointed
wings, etc., they do not often remain in the eye, for they
soon become covered with mucus and slip out. It is surprising to see how rapidly the mucus collects around
such objects; in a few minutes a little fly will be all
gummed up. Has not the reader noticed, when a single
eyelash is removed from behind the lower lid, how it is
buried in sticky mucus? That the larvæ of certain
insects can reach the conjunctiva is shown by the following case:

A negro from the Indian Territory was admitted
to the City Hospital suffering from severe inflammation
of the nose, eyes, and head. The man was in a dreadful condition. The pain had almost worn him out.
There was great swelling of the face and almost com-

plete closure of the nose from œdema of the mucous membrane. I found that all the sinuses in his head were filled with the larvæ of the Texas fly. In examining his eyes, I discovered a large maggot free on the conjunctiva and another working its way out of the lachrymal sac. They were removed. The man was cured by filling his nose with the vapor of chloroform, then syringing it out with dilute creolin. It was several weeks before all traces of the larvæ disappeared.

The annoyance and pain excited by a foreign body will depend largely upon its position, size, and character. They all irritate more or less, but a piece of straw or wood may remain for a long time imprisoned in the folds of the upper cul-de-sac and be unnoticed.

Small cinders adhering to the lid do not worry the individual unless they come in contact with the cornea; then the pain may be very severe, and if the offending particle is not removed, an inflammation may be excited very much like acute catarrh. Little pieces of stone, steel, metal of any kind, or grains of powder sticking on or in the cornea will always cause trouble if they remain over a few hours. Because, in these instances, the irritation is confined alone to the cornea, the congestion affects principally the ciliary vessels, as in iritis or keratitis. Then there is a rose-colored zone around the circumference of the cornea; the pupil will be contracted, also photophobia and lachrymation. In these cases the severity of the symptoms is nearly always dependent upon the size of the object. Large cinders buried in the cornea excite a great deal of inflammation; small ones, on or under the surface, irritate from time to time. The individual will congratulate himself often during the day that it is out, to be disappointed at night, when he attempts to read.

Minute particles of emery or steel on the cornea invariably excite great irritation in the eye.   So much so, that, if the doctor is not careful, he may overlook the cause and treat for iritis.   The same with poder-grains.   The little sharp hairs from certain plants and off some caterpillars excite great disturbance in the eye if they reach the conjunctiva.   The cause is mechanical and chemical, so one can picture the condition that can be excited by them.

The only danger to be feared from foreign bodies is acute keratitis, but that is remote, for the patient will use every possible means to have the offending material removed.   Again let me assure the reader that if there is a chronic purulent inflammation of the lachrymal sac, the simplest wound of the cornea which opens into the lymphatic spaces may lead to destruction of the eye, from septic infection.

Diagnosis.—Although, as a rule, the diagnosis—a foreign body, is easy when the foreign body can be seen, still it is sometimes very difficult, for one cannot always readily find it.   An expert will in the majority of cases make a correct diagnosis from the general appearance of the eye, but a doctor who has not had much experi-ence in such cases may be puzzled to know what is the matter.

If a patient complains of something in the eye and it is not found on the upper lid when it is turned, the probabilities are it is on the cornea and will be seen if the eye is examined through a watchmaker's glass. Even then it is sometimes necessary to use focal illumination, especially if the injury is received at the emery-wheel. If an eye is badly inflamed 24 hours after a gunpowder accident and it is not burnt, the trouble is in the cornea. Powder wounds of the con-junctiva do not pain much. In cases of monocular blennorrhœa without disease of the lachrymal sac ex-amine carefully for a foreign body. Turn the upper lid and, by the method already given, spring the retro-tarsal folds in view; search carefully the cul-de-sac. If there are granulations (proud flesh), the great prob-ability is there is an irritating substance buried in the tissues. The probe and forceps should soon settle the question. The practitioner should never neglect the retrotarsal folds in such cases. Children may require an anæsthetic.

Treatment.—There is but one treatment: Remove the foreign body if it can be done. Powder-grains in and under the conjunctiva cannot be removed. Many of them will break down and be partly absorbed; the rest will remain for life. A very large powder-grain distinctly elevating the membrane may be grasped with a pair of forceps and cut away, together with a piece of the conjunctiva. If the wound gaps very much, a single stitch may be advisable; otherwise it will heal promptly without a perceptible scar. A foreign body sticking to the cornea is best removed by passing over it a piece of absorbent cotton wrapped around the end of a probe. It will usually be caught in the meshes of the cotton and pulled off. If that is not successful, it is best to benumb the cornea with cocaine and then pick it off with an appropriate instrument. A body

buried in the superficial layers of the cornea is best
picked out with a cataract-needle. But the operation
should be done under a glass, for often more of the
cornea is picked to pieces than is necessary. It is difficult to remove pieces of emery, especially if they are
minute. When a piece of iron or steel sticks on the
cornea and remains a day or so, it oxidizes and deeply
stains the tissues immediately around. After the body
is removed from its bed, it will be found that a little
dark ring is left. This deposit is as irritating as the
body itself, and should be removed. It is best done by
paring it off with a sharp needle. The ease with which
a foreign body is removed will depend very much upon
the tension of the eye. Cocaine, if used for any length
of time, will make the eye very soft, when it may be
impossible to use a needle successfully; so it is advisable, if the object is not removed before the eye grows
soft, to wait a few hours and try again. The after-
treatment is simple. When the cornea is injured after
removing a foreign body, the eye should be washed with
a mild antiseptic (boracic acid solution), then bandaged
for a few hours. If there is pain, a drop of a 0.5 per
cent solution of homatropine will be soothing. Atropia relieves instantly, but its after-effect prohibits its
use, unless the reactive inflammation is so severe that
its employment is imperative. Often the patient will
return and complain that the foreign body is not out;
sometimes it is not, but usually the sandy feeling, in
such instances, is dependent upon the same cause as it
is in catarrhal ophthalmia.

BURNS.

The conjunctiva can be burnt by flame, hot bodies, steam, chemical substance, and the rays from the arc-electric light. Like on the skin, these burns are graded from simple irritation to complete destruction of the mucous membrane. The simplest burn is the common sun burn, which never happens from the direct rays, but from the reflected ones. It is mostly seen in amateur fishermen. It will be noticed that those who suffer from severe sun dermatitis of the face often have red, congested eyes. The same is seen in mountain-climbers and adventurers of the North, the sun's rays being reflected from the snow. Burns of this kind are excited by the rays coming from the arc electric light. In these cases the symptoms are very severe; there is not only severe dermatitis and swelling of the face and lids, but also œdema and inflammation of the conjunctiva very much like acute catarrh. The eye-pain and the photophobia are distressing. Workmen about electric furnaces and welding machinery are subject to it. Steam burns of the conjunctiva are not uncommon. Of course, the severity of the burn will depend upon the heat of the steam and its tension. Such accidents usually occur about boiler explosions and in railroad wrecks. If the steam escapes from a ruptured boiler or pipe, it will burn the conjunctiva before the lids can be closed. Such burns of the conjunctiva are not apt to be very severe; usually there is congestion of the eye and exfoliation of the corneal epithelium.

Those caught in illuminating gas explosions are always burnt about the eyes. The flame, which is very hot, reaches the conjunctiva before the lids close, because the reflex action from the retina to the orbicularis muscles is too slow to protect the eye. All burns of that kind I have seen were subjectively severe, but the eyes were not permanently damaged. If in gunpowder accidents the eyes are destroyed, the flame is rarely responsible, for it does not remain long enough in contact with the conjunctiva to sphacelate it. The damage is usually done by the force of the explosion or the foreign bodies driven against the eye. Lighted cigars and cigarettes burn the eye dreadfully when they touch it. Parlor-match burns are very severe, because the fire does not go out immediately. Glowing cinders and molten metal always destroy the area of the conjunctiva they touch. Such burns are usually on the under half of the eye or in the lower cul-de-sac.

The most common chemical burns are from lime, ammonia, and acids. Lime burns are of two kinds: those made by slacked and unslacked lime. Really they are the same burns, but differ in degree. It is not often that a person gets sufficient pure lime in the eyes to damage them; but should such an accident occur, the conjunctiva would be certainly destroyed and the cornea rendered permanently opaque. Lime burns usually occur when a quantity of fresh mortar strikes the eye, which often happens to workmen looking up from the basement of a building. The mortar then hits the open eye with considerable force, and, as a rule, fills the conjunctival sac with sand and partly slacked lime. That generally injures the mucous membrane, but the greatest damage is done the cornea. Al-

most immediately the alkali penetrates to the superficial layers, and either destroys them or renders them
opaque. The corneal epithelium always turns white.
The pain from the sand and chemical is very severe; so
much so that the physician may have great difficulty in
cleaning the eye.

Since the introduction of ice-making machines in the
cities and nearly all large towns, ammonia burns are
becoming quite common. They are usually severe and
excite considerable inflammation, but I have never seen
the eye destroyed by that means. It can happen, for
liquid anhydrous ammonia is used, and that will immediately kill living tissues.

Pure sulphuric and nitric acids destroy immediately
all the mucous surfaces they reach. They, too, turn the
cornea white. The subjective symptoms are severe.
These accidents rarely happen to the eye alone. The
skin of the lids is usually cauterized. Indeed, the
greatest danger is to be feared from the consequent
deformity of the lids. Dilute acids usually fly into the
eye in explosions of chemical apparatus. The parts
may be severely burned, but it is not the rule that the
eye is damaged so much from the chemical as from the
flying pieces of the retort.

Treatment.—In simple burns of the conjunctiva,
when there is hyperæmia and loss of the corneal epithelium, it is well to anoint the inside of the lids with vaseline, instill atropia, and apply cold compresses. Unfortunately, little more can be done for severe burns. We
must wait until the sloughs come away, then try and
hasten the healing. If two opposing conjunctival ulcers meet at the cul-de-sac, nothing will prevent the lid

and eye-ball growing together.   The doctor may try by
separating them, and congratulate himself that he has
succeeded, but in the end he will be disappointed.   The
lid will adhere to the eyeball over the burnt area.
Therefore it is best to let Nature take her course, hop-
ing that a plastic operation may remedy the deformity.
The best treatment for severe, deep burns of the cornea
is atropia and a compress bandage.   When the conjunctiva is burnt by molten metal, the great difficulty
will be to remove the foreign bodies, because often the
metal will be adhering tightly to the mucosa.

Lime burns are annoying to treat.   In the first
place, the physician must give a prognosis, and it may
be several days before he can determine how much of
the conjunctiva is destroyed.   If the cornea is not dry
and the iris can be, even faintly, seen, the probabilities
are that the white cloud will disappear.   If, on the
other hand, the opacity is so dense that nothing back
of the cornea is visible, the chances are that the eye
is ruined.   There is no certainty, however, unless the
cornea is dead; otherwise it is advisable to be guarded
in the prognosis.   Some of the most desperately burnt
eyes will recover in a way that is surprising.

It is not often the physician has an opportunity to
see a case immediately after chemical burns of the eye.
Acids are very rapidly neutralized by the copious flow
of tears they excite, and liquid alkalies are soon washed
out.   If, however, the doctor is present at the accident,
the best he can do is to wash out the conjunctival sac
thoroughly with plain water.   It takes time to prepare
chemical antidotes; water is always handy and effect-

ive. When a piece of solid but melting chemical is caught under the lids, such as a crystal of the nitrate of silver or a lump of unslacked lime, he should not attempt to wash it out, but turn the lids and remove it. Water will invariably make the bad worse. If the burn is severe, the eye is to be filled with pure vaseline or olive oil and cold compresses applied. That is all that can be done for the time being. The after-effects must be treated on general surgical principles. Should a child get some freshly slacked lime in its eyes, the conjunctival sac may be washed out with olive or sweet oil, which is the best mechanical and chemical antidote.

When an eye is filled with mortar, the lids must be turned, and the eye cleaned with a piece of cotton cloth; then it should be cocainized, and every piece of sand removed, which will surely be found sticking to the lids and eyeball; finally, the conjunctival sac must be filled with dilute sugar syrup (Von Arlt), then a cold compress applied. In these cases the doctor should be careful in making a positive prognosis, for it may be several hours before the full effect of the injury can be appreciated.

Simple wounds of the conjunctiva are usually trivial affairs, for it is very seldom the mucous membrane is so badly torn that stitching is necessary. Then, usually, the eye itself is damaged. Small wounds heal very rapidly without a scar. Even a few hours after a foreign body has penetrated the sclera, it is often hard to find where it pierced the conjunctiva. Extensive wounds may close up rapidly. For example, a man was brought into the hospital, comatose. A day or so before

—11—

he had fallen on a pick; at that time his eye bled some. When I saw him, it was evident that he had some cerebral lesion, although it was impossible to find where it was. At first I could not see that the eye was injured, nor could I by probing the cul-de-sacs find any hole such as a pick would make. Finally I found that the point of the pick had glanced off the cornea, penetrated the conjunctiva at the corneal edge, and, passing between it and the eyeball, punctured the roof of the orbit. The eye was enucleated, the orbit cleaned out, and a large quantity of broken-down brain-matter and bone removed. The man recovered. This case was under the care of Dr. King at the Missouri Pacific Hospital in this city. It is cited to show that a very extensive wound of the conjunctiva may escape the scrutiny of trained observers. Usually, conjunctival wounds are best let alone; when, however, they gape, it is well to bring the edges together with a stitch to avoid healing by second intention and the growth of granulations.

HEMORRHAGE.

A very common accident is hemorrhage under the conjunctiva. Sometimes this is a matter of no moment; at other times it is a very serious symptom, especially if it follows a head injury.

Often a blood-vessel will break behind the conjunctiva, and in a few minutes the eyeball will become blood-red. Usually the hemorrhage is diffused over a large part of the eye, rarely over all. When the blood reaches the cornea, it stops advancing, but in a few hours the coloring matter will enter the eyeball and stain the iris. Because of gravity, the mass of blood sinks to the lower cul-de-sac, and may reach the conjunctiva of the lids. It is not often there is enough blood to make a distinct bleb; usually it is only a deep stain.

This condition is always very alarming to the patient, for, as a rule, his attention is first called to it by his friends. The looking-glass is consulted, and immediately afterwards the doctor. Now, although this is often a trivial affair, still it demands of the doctor the most careful study. From no apparent reason, a blood-vessel has given way. The same could happen in the brain and be of serious moment. Consequently he should hunt for the cause. It may be a slight trauma, or straining at stool. Never turn these cases away with the promise that all will be well, without first examining the urine. Be sure there is not Bright's disease or diabetes. In fracture of the skull, either of the vault or base, subconjunctival hemorrhage is diagnostic, especially in wounds of the side of the head with rupture of the middle meningeal artery; but simple blows on the temple, like fist-blows on the eye, are often followed by ecchymosis of the eyeball, irrespective of fracture or dangerous injury. The best treatment is to leave the parts alone. If the eye is seen at the beginning of the bleeding, a compress bandage may stop it. In severe hemorrhage with bulging of the conjunctiva an incision to let out the superfluous blood is advisable, but the wound must be treated antiseptically.

Ordinarily the blood will be absorbed in from two to six weeks, and it may leave a faint stain on the sclera for months.

INDEX.

15 ①

www.ingramcontent.com/pod-product-compliance
Lightning Source LLC
Chambersburg PA
CBHW021704210326
41599CB00013B/1518